3/06

the Abs Diet Get Fit, Stay Fit Plan

The Exercise Program to Flatten Your Belly, Reshape Your Body, and Give You Abs for Life!

DAVID ZINCZENKO, *Editor-in-Chief of* **Men'sHealth.**

WITH TED SPIKER

© 2006 by Rodale Inc.

Exercise photographs © 2006 by Beth Bischoff
"'Thanks, Abs Diet!'" photographs courtesy of respective photograph subjects

Printed in the United States of America

Rodale Inc. makes every effort to use acid-free ♾, recycled paper ♻.

Book design by Christopher Rhoads
Exercise photos by Beth Bischoff

Library of Congress Cataloging-in-Publication Data

Zinczenko, David.
    The abs diet get fit, stay fit plan : the exercise plan to flatten your belly, reshape your body, and give you abs for life! / David Zinczenko with Ted Spiker.
        p.   cm.
    Includes index.
    ISBN-13 978–1–59486–409–4 hardcover
    ISBN-10 1–59486–409–8 hardcover
    1. Exercise for men.   2. Physical fitness for men.   3. Abdomen—Muscles.   4. Reducing diets.
5. Nutrition.   6. Men—Health and hygiene.   I. Spiker, Ted.   II. Title.
RA781.Z56 2006
613.7—dc22   2005026004

Distributed to the trade by Holtzbrinck Publishers

2   4   6   8   10   9   7   5   3   1   hardcover

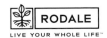

LIVE YOUR WHOLE LIFE™

We inspire and enable people to improve their lives and the world around them

For more of our products visit **rodalestore.com** or call 800-848-4735

www.theAbsDiet.com

This book is dedicated to Ronald McDonald (you clown!), Burger King, the Taco Bell Chihuahua, Bob the Quiznos baby, and all the other characters out there whose job it's been to sell us fast food at a tender young age. We're not swallowing your junk anymore!

Contents

Acknowledgments

Seeing the *Abs Diet* and the *Get Fit, Stay Fit Plan* come to fruition has been one of the great pleasures of my life. Seeing it make a real impact on the lives of tens of thousands of Americans has been one of the great rewards. For all of it, I have to thank a number of extraordinarily talented, hard-working, and dedicated people who continue to support, encourage, and inspire me. In particular:

Steve Murphy, whose courage and commitment to editorial quality has made Rodale Inc. the best publishing company in the world for which to work.

The Rodale family, without whom none of this would be possible.

Ben Roter, whom I want to be when I grow up.

Ted Spiker, the world's best coauthor.

Steve Perrine, who works his creative magic day in and day out.

The entire *Men's Health* editorial staff, the smartest and hardest-working group of writers, editors, researchers, designers, and photo directors in the industry. A big shout-out to Rob Gerth, Myatt Murphy, Beth Bischoff, Kathryn C. LeSage, Chris Krogermeier, Chris Rhoads, Kelly Schmidt, Hope Clarke, Nancy Bailey, Karen Neely, Emily Williams, Keith Biery, Wendy Hess, Jennifer Giandomenico, Brenda Miller, David Umla, and everyone else who worked so hard and so fast to publish this book.

My brother, Eric, whose relentless teasing shamed me into taking better care of myself. (Dude, you're sooo dead. . . .)

My mother, Janice, who raised two of us nearly single-handedly. Your strength and kindness guide my every action.

My dad, Bohdan, who left this world way too early. I wish you were still here.

My uncle, Denny Stanz, the picture of youthfulness.

My stepmother, Mickey, ditto.

Elaine Kaufman, who still lets me order off the menu.

And special thanks to: Dan Abrams, Jeff Anthony, Mary Ann Bekkedahl, Tami Booth Corwin, Michael Bruno, Adam Campbell, Jeff Csatari, Kimberly Guilfoyle Newsom, Jon

Hammond and Karen Mazzotta, Joe Heroun, Erin Hobday, Samantha Irwin, George Karabotsos, Charlene Lutz, MM and RP!, Vincent Maggio, Patrick McMullan, Peter Moore, Jeff Morgan, Sarah Peters, Bill Phillips, Scott Quill, Phillip Rhodes, Leslie Schneider, Zachary Schisgal, Joyce Shirer, Bill Stump, John Tayman, Pat and Steve Toomey, and Sara Vigneri. Thanks for all the rock-solid advice. You guys rule.

TIME FOR A CHANGE

You Have to Make Up Your Mind If You Want to Make Over Your Body

CHANGE, THEY SAY, IS GOOD FOR US.

But like most everything else that's good for us—cough medicine, fiber supplements, the programming on PBS—change can sometimes be a little hard to choke down. The grown-up world is an unsettling place, and when we find a comfort zone—in our jobs, in our relationships, or in our sofas and easy chairs—we like to stay there.

But the most comfortable place isn't always the healthiest place.

Sixty-two percent of Americans today are overweight or obese. And most of us who struggle with our weight would like to make a change. But change has always been hard.

Until now.

When I developed the Abs Diet in 2004, I did it with that very thing in mind: I wanted people to change. I wanted to start a program that would inspire people to eat better, live healthier, be leaner, and develop stomachs flatter than a plasma screen TV. And that's really what the Abs Diet is all about. It's about changing the way you eat, and the way you think about nutrition and exercise. It's about changing your body—and your health.

And here's the amazing part: It's easy.

If you read the success stories of the people featured in this book—as well as the original *Abs Diet* and *The Abs Diet Eat Right Every Time Guide*—you'll find one common theme. The people who lose fat with the Abs Diet say it isn't a diet. It's a change in philosophy, a change in lifestyle, a change in a healthier, leaner direction. I've read the stories of so many men and women who've written to tell me how the Abs Diet has changed their lives: contributing more energy, lower cholesterol numbers, smaller pants, and a more powerful sex drive. The Abs Diet is not only changing America's bodies—it's changing our lives.

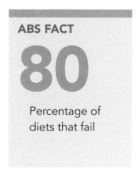

ABS FACT

80

Percentage of
diets that fail

What most people find so amazing about the Abs Diet is its simple nutritional principles. The Abs Diet is built around 12 delicious food groups—I call them the Powerfoods.

These 12 Powerfoods will make you over faster than those guys from Queer Eye. (You can read more about the principles of the Abs Diet and how the Powerfoods will work for you by turning to Chapter 5 of this book.) But the right diet is only so effective. If you truly want to make over your body and your life—if you truly want change—you need to unleash your body's real potential with the secret ingredient found in this book: exercise.

Now, hold on, hold on. Remember what I said at the beginning of this chapter: Change is good, but sometimes it seems hard. Well, listen, while the idea of changing your body through exercise *seems* hard, it isn't—at least, not when you incorporate the principles of the Abs Diet Get Fit, Stay Fit Plan.

For example, I bet the first thing you thought when I mentioned exercise was, "I have to burn off calories in the gym." Well, guess what? You're wrong. The Abs Diet Get Fit, Stay Fit Plan isn't about burning calories in the gym. In fact, let's go back to that comfort zone, the sofa, the easy chair. How would you like to burn off life-altering quantities of calories *while you're lounging in your recliner*? Or, how about while you're lying in bed? Driving your car? Checking your e-mail? Eating?

That's what this plan is designed to do: to train your body to burn calories all the time, everywhere, even while you're at rest—heck, even while you're asleep. The key is to reset your body's metabolism, to teach it to burn more calories, all the time, not just when you exercise. And you do that by building muscle. Not governor-of-California muscle. Not Rambo-covered-with-leeches muscle. Just lean, firm, powerful muscle that fights fat even while keeping your body safe from injury.

How can building muscle actually fight fat? It's simple: For every pound of muscle you build, your body needs to burn an extra 50 calories a day just to maintain itself. So even a modest increase of three pounds of muscle means another 150 calories a day you're burning just by sitting around, staring at the walls, pondering the big questions like "What is the nature of God?" and "Why is Paris Hilton famous?"

In *The Abs Diet*, I presented the Abs Diet Workout, a program to reshape your body and replace unsightly flab with lean, healthy muscle. And the workout has been a phenomenon, spawning videos, magazine articles, and even a Web site that attracts loyal adherents who have seen their bodies change almost effortlessly—and who want to share their success stories with others.

But all workout programs—even the very best of them—are like those little tape recorders Mr. Phelps used to listen to at the beginning of *Mission: Impossible*. Even the very best workout plans are designed to self-destruct—maybe not after five seconds, but after five weeks or so, definitely.

That's because our bodies are incredibly adept at adjusting to the demands we place on them. Like toddlers, our bodies learn and adapt. And when we exercise using the same routine day in and day out, our bodies adapt too. Over time, we begin to lose the benefits of even the best workout program, simply because our muscles are like Bill Clinton: They mean well, but they just can't help cheating.

And that's why I wrote this book. I wanted those who had already seen tremendous success with the Abs Diet to keep improving, to keep reshaping their bodies the way they wanted. And I wanted those who were new to the Abs Diet to have a head start, to have at their fingertips a whole collection of easy, effective exercises.

With hundreds of exercises, I want this guide to serve as your ultimate training manual. You'll be equipped to develop many different Abs Diet training programs. Best of all, I've given you options no matter what your situation—whether you belong to a gym or work out at home, whether you lift dumbbells or Junior, whether you have to exercise in a hotel room or cell block H. Even with thousands of exercise combinations, there's one thing that won't change when it comes to the Abs Diet Workout: that's the overarching principle about how to build your body and flatten your stomach so that throughout your life you can continually challenge your muscles and keep your body in the best possible shape. In short, the Abs Diet Workout system has its foundation in this acronym:

ABS FACT

30

Percentage more sex had by men who exercise 3 days a week

ABS3

The ABS3 system works because it allows you to put emphasis on the kinds of exercise that research has shown to be effective for speeding metabolism, burning fat, and building muscle. The book details how the principle works, shows dozens of different programs that you can immediately start using, and gives you the tools to mix and match exercises so that you can do what we're all wired to do: Keep changing. In short, ABS3 stands for:

A = Abdominal muscles. You'll work your abdominal muscles two or three times a week to develop a strong, lean, flat, 6-pack core of muscles.

B = Big muscle groups. You'll do strength-training that emphasizes the largest muscles in your body because those are the muscles that best help you burn fat.

S = Speed intervals. Interval training (cardiovascular work that mixes high-intensity effort with low-intensity effort) has been shown to be more effective for losing fat than steady-state cardiovascular exercise.

3 = 3 times per week. You can achieve results in just three workouts a week.

Woody Allen once said that 90 percent of success is just showing up. That's probably not true for most things in life, but when it comes to the Abs Diet Get Fit, Stay Fit Plan, Woody's philosophy actually holds true. The program is so easy, all you have to do is make time for it.

But, ah, there's the rub: making time for it. That's why I've designed this program to be completed in just three sessions of 20 minutes each. Sixty total minutes a week—if you can find time to watch an episode of *Desperate Housewives*, you can find time for this.

And make no mistake, though it may seem to take no time at all, your results from this program will be dramatic.

I'll go into depth about the ABS3 plan a little later in the book. But before I do, I want to tell you a little bit about how I view exercise—and why I truly believe that anyone can use it to reshape their body and recharge their life.

See, I didn't grow up as some star athlete or superfit aerobics addict. I was an overweight kid who spent more time watching sports than playing them. I was so fat and sloppy that when I finally did get involved in sports by joining the wrestling team, the coach used me as the "stopper"—essentially, I would go into the ring and just flop down on top of my opponent until the buzzer rang. I wasn't really a wrestler. I was a 200-pound bag of suet with a jock strap.

Then I graduated high school (early photos of what scientists believed to be a black hole were, in fact, pictures of me in a graduation gown) and joined the Naval Reserves. Suddenly, things changed. For the first time in my life, I was made to exercise. And the pounds came off. When I left the Navy, I joined *Men's Health* magazine, where I learned even more about the importance of fitness and made it a permanent part of my life. Today, my career is dedicated to helping people live healthy, active lives. Exercise fends

ABS FACT

80

Percent of every pound that you lose that's fat, if you're exercising regularly off diseases from diabetes to stroke to heart disease; prevents injuries and osteoporosis; increases your energy while diminishing your stress; and inspires your sex drive (and the sex drives of those around you). And if better health, a longer life, a sexier body, and a stress-proof existence sounds good to you . . . well, the chance for change is now. Seize it.

Now, you might be thinking to yourself, "This guy works for *Men's Health*. He gets paid to curl dumbbells with one hand while typing out e-mails with the other. *Of course* he has time to exercise." Well, I have one word for you: baloney (which, you'll discover, is *not* a Powerfood.)

My philosophy is that exercise can't be like a jealous boyfriend or girlfriend—high-maintenance and more trouble than it's worth. It has to be like the perfect partner in that it complements the rest of your life. Otherwise, there's no incentive to keep to the program, and you'll just end up breaking up with it in the long run.

I know all the obstacles to getting into a regular exercise routine. You have a job. You have overtime. You have a schedule. You have family. You have a couch that swallows you as soon as you sit down. You have Jimmy the toddler hanging off one arm and JoJo the terrier tugging on the other. You have lots of reasons *not* to exercise. But the Abs Diet is a program that anyone can do, because it's one that you can do at the gym, at home, with equipment, without equipment. Whatever your lifestyle, you can employ the ABS3 principles.

> **ABS FACT**
>
> # 60
>
> Percentage of men and women who want toned abs more than any other muscular trait

I'll leave you with this one last thought. I wish people would stop thinking of exercise like it's scrubbing tile. Sure, in the beginning, it can feel like hard work; it can feel like a chore. But I want you to think of exercise as a little bit like merging onto an interstate. Yes, it's going to take you a little gas to build up some steam, and you may hit a curve here and there as you get going. But once you accelerate into a program, once you find your groove, once you start seeing results, you'll be on exercise cruise control. That's because it's much easier to maintain good fitness with regular workouts than it is to get there in the first place. And that's what helps trigger the cycle of lean living. Once you're able to teach your body to speed your metabolism—through the proper food and exercise—you'll teach it to burn fat all day. And that's really our goal, isn't it?

Get fit.

Stay fit.

Live fit.

Do those three things, and you'll reach your ultimate destination: Pants fit.

THE FLAT-BELLY TEST

How close are you to the stomach you've always wanted?

So what if the last test you took was of the paternity variety; you can fly through this one, which will gauge your potential for developing a flat stomach and a 6-pack. Don't worry if your score plunges lower than Mariah Carey's neckline. Follow the ABS3 principles and Abs Diet Workout for 6 weeks, then take the test again—and see how far you've come.

Add up your total points.

AGE

Your metabolism slows with age. The older you get, the less fat you burn at rest.

Younger than 25	+2
25–35	+1
Older than 35	-1

BODY FAT

The higher your fat level, the longer it'll take to see your abs (see "Size Yourself Up" on page 4 for instructions on determining your body fat percentage).

Below 10 percent	+2
10–15 percent	+1
Higher than 15 percent	-1

MOTIVATION

If you skip workouts regularly, you won't make as much progress.

Consistently work out 3 or more times per week	+2
2 times per week	+1
Fewer than 2 times per week	-1

DIET

High amounts of bad-for-you fat will derail your program.

Less than 30 percent of daily calories from fat	+1
30 percent or more of daily calories from fat	-1

WEIGHT LIFTING

Strength training is proven to help raise your metabolism and build muscle mass, including the abdominals.

Strength training with challenging weights 3 or more times per week	+2
Light weights 3 or more times per week	+1
No weight training	-1

INTERVAL TRAINING

Sprinting is a high-intensity workout, burning more calories and raising metabolism.

At least one interval session per week	+2
No intervals	0

WALKING/CARDIO

Walking or doing light steady cardio exercise at least 2 days a week	+2
Doing less than 2 days a week	0

STRESS

High levels of the stress hormone cortisol may make you pack on abdominal fat.

Low stress	+1
Some stress	0
High stress	-1

CRUNCHES

The classic ab exercise, but doing too many too often can work against you.

2 or 3 crunch sessions per week	+1
Crunch infrequently	0
No crunching	-1
More than 3 sessions per week	-1

YOUR SCORE

8 points or higher: On your way to a 6-pack, if you're not there already.

3–7: Getting close

2 or lower: Gut may look like the beer truck instead.

THE ABS DIET CHEAT SHEET

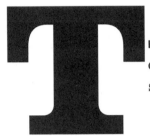**HIS AT-A-GLANCE GUIDE** summarizes the principles of the Abs Diet: the 6-week plan to flatten your stomach and keep you lean for life.

EXERCISE

The ABS3 exercise program is optional for the first 2 weeks. Base your plan around these components for the most effective fat-burning plan.

A = Abdominal muscles

B = Big muscle groups (strength training)

S = Speed intervals (high-intensity cardiovascular exercise mixed with periods of low-intensity)

3 = 3x/week

At-home workout	Gym workouts and at-home workouts are both detailed to excuse-proof your fitness plan.
Abdominal workout	At the beginning of two of your strength-training workouts. One exercise for each of the five different parts of your abs.

DIET

SUBJECT	GUIDELINE
Number of meals	Six a day, spaced relatively evenly throughout the day. Eat snacks 2 hours before larger meals.

SUBJECT	GUIDELINE
The **ABS DIET POWER 12**	Base most of your meals on these 12 groups of foods. Every meal should have at least two foods from the list.
	Almonds and other nuts
	Beans and legumes
	Spinach and other green vegetables
	Dairy (fat-free or low-fat milk, yogurt, cheese)
	Instant oatmeal (unsweetened, unflavored)
	Eggs
	Turkey and other lean meats
	Peanut butter
	Olive oil
	Whole-grain breads and cereals
	Extra-protein (whey) powder
	Raspberries and other berries
Secret weapons	Each of the ABS DIET POWER 12 has been chosen in part for its stealthy, healthy secret weapons—the nutrients that will help power up your natural fat burners, protect you from illness and injury, and keep you lean and fit for life!
Nutritional ingredients to emphasize	Protein, monounsaturated and polyunsaturated fats, fiber, calcium.
Nutritional ingredients to limit	Refined carbohydrates (or carbs with high glycemic index), saturated fats, trans fats, high-fructose corn syrup.
Alcohol	Limit yourself to two or three drinks per week, to maximize the benefits of the Abs Diet plan.
Ultimate power food	Smoothies. The calcium and protein in milk, yogurt, and whey powder combined with the fiber in oatmeal and fruit makes them one of the easier and more satisfying options in the diet. Drink them regularly.
Portion control	There's no counting calories, measuring food, or weighing portions. Focusing on the Power 12 foods should regulate your hunger so that you don't feel the need to have big portions. Still, it's always smart to have reasonable portions—that is, cover your plate with good proteins, grains, vegetables, and healthy fat, but remember that a height restriction is in effect.
Cheating	One meal a week, eat anything you want.

Chapter I

ABS3: THE ULTIMATE EXERCISE PLAN

The Equation for a Lean, Fit, and Strong Body Lies in These Three Factors

IN HEALTH CIRCLES, everyone talks about the obesity epidemic. We're a fat society. We eat too much. We eat badly. We deep-fry perfectly good vegetables, for God's sake. And it's one of the main reasons we're a country with bellies the size of Jupiter. But there's something lost in all the talk about creamy sauces, grease-laced buffets, super-sized fries, and exotic coffee drinks that are the caloric equivalents of Big Macs. We're not just in an obesity epidemic. We're in an inactivity epidemic.

A recent study by the National Center for Health Statistics found that only 19 percent of the population regularly engages in "high levels of physical activity." And by "high levels", they mean only 1 hour per week. That means 4 out of 5 of us aren't getting the amount of exercise we need. (And consider this: 1 hour a week is just 1 percent of the time you're awake every week.) Now, the problem isn't that we don't know what we need to do. In fact, 63 percent of Americans—about the same percentage who are

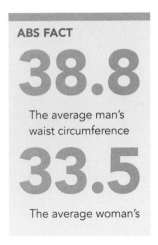

ABS FACT

38.8

The average man's
waist circumference

33.5

The average woman's

overweight—believe that exercise would help them live healthier and leaner. What we need is a plan that really works—without really feeling like work.

Having worked at *Men's Health* magazine for more than 10 years, I've seen more dumbbells than an *American Idol* tryout. I've seen all the trends (uh, electrodes on my abs, no thanks). I've talked to trainers. I've tried hundreds of exercises. In a lot of ways, my workout is part of my work. But I also know what it's like to be slammed with calls, meetings, writing e-mails, and all of the daily stresses and responsibilities that go into any job. So I know exactly what you want out of an exercise plan: You want a program that *fits* into your life—not one that *is* your life.

That's why I've constructed ABS3: to help you burn fat at the highest levels possible in the least amount of time. I want this plan to be flexible and convenient—an excuse-proof program that gives you the tools to work it around any schedule. My overriding philosophy: Keep the workout short and keep it simple, and you'll stay focused and motivated. Oh, you'll work up a sweat and you'll breathe heavier than a 900-number operator. That's the only way you'll see results—by challenging your body. But you won't have to claim squatter's rights at the gym to do so. Ab for ab, it's the best workout to flatten your stomach, lose fat, build muscle, and change your body forever.

A = Abdominal Muscles

Abs are a little like distant cousins. Everybody has them, but hardly anybody ever really gets to see them—or even remembers what they look like. Typically, that's because ab muscles are smothered in a layer of belly fat called visceral fat. It's the most dangerous fat there is because of its proximity to your body's organs. So, one order of business is to remove it. That does *not* happen with abdominal exercises. That happens with diet, with training your big muscle groups (the B in ABS3), and with the speed interval training (the S).

So, can't we just skip the ab work? Uh-uh. You've still got to crunch away like a CPA in April. By working your abdominal muscles twice a week, you'll build them so that when you do burn fat, your abs will, in fact, stand out like Michael Moore at a GOP meeting. But

LET'S GET IT STARTED

An exercise novice? Follow these rules for an easy transition into ABS3

If you're new to strength training, the biggest mistake you can make is jumping in head first. Exercise doesn't have to be intimidating, but if you rush into it, you'll increase your chance of failing by becoming too frustrated, too tired, too sore, too overwhelmed. Instead, follow these guidelines:

• **Get the food figured out first.** If you're just starting the Abs Diet, it's not critical that that you start working out immediately. Concentrate on acclimating your body to eating the Powerfoods six times a day to fuel your body. That fuel will be what gives you energy for the day, as well as for your workout. Take 2 weeks with diet only, and then add the exercise program.

• **Start light.** If you do want to start a light strength-training program immediately, do this workout three times a week: Alternate between three sets of pushups and three sets of squats with no weight. Both exercises use your body weight as resistance and will get your body accustomed to a strength-training program. Do 8 to 10 repetitions of pushups, followed by 15 to 20 repetitions of squats. When that becomes too easy, increase the repetitions of pushups and hold on to some form of weight—light dumbbells are best—while doing squats. This light workout, especially in combination with 30 minutes of brisk walking, will really fire up your fat burners.

• **Start small, grow stronger.** If the only time you've ever picked up a dumbbell was that unfortunate weekend in Vegas, don't go off and start playing Hercules right away. You can start by lifting any amount of weight that you're comfortable with—whether it's a pair of light dumbbells, a couple of cans of beans, or the lightest notch on the weight machine. Even if you start small, you'll grow stronger, begin to build muscle, and keep your metabolism revved. As you progress, you'll build and burn more. Light weights give you an opportunity to master the form before trying to do exercises with a challenging amount of resistance.

even more importantly, abdominal exercises help you build a center of strength that not only turns heads but also makes you healthier. For example, gaining strength in your core—that is, your entire trunk, not just the visible 6-pack muscles in the front—has more benefits than a CEO's annual contract. Maybe the most convincing data is this: In a recent Canadian study of more than 8,000 people, researchers found that over 13 years, those with the weakest abdominal muscles had a death rate more than twice as high as that of those with the strongest midsections. Pretty amazing, huh? Of course, there's a very strong link between smaller waist sizes and better health; in short, when you develop your abs and strip away fat, you make your entire body healthier—by reducing your risk of everything from heart disease to diabetes. (And that's not to mention that having a strong midsection has also been shown to improve your sex life because less fat helps improve blood flow, which is important for both male and female sexual satisfaction.) But just in case improving your health, your looks, and your sex life isn't enough for you, developing your core strength with abdominal exercises has many other benefits, such as the following:

Abs protect you. A U.S. Army study linked powerful abdominal muscles to injury prevention. After giving 120 artillery soldiers the standard army fitness test of situps, pushups, and a 2-mile run, researchers tracked their lower-body injuries (such as lower-

SIZE YOURSELF UP

The best way to keep track of your progress is by taking a few key measurements

When you're winning at the craps table, you keep rolling. And when you're winning in an exercise program, you keep rolling. Seeing results—whether it's in pounds, inches, or body fat percentage—can be one of your best motivators. I recommend taking readings of key measurements every 2 weeks. That's enough distance so you'll see some results, but not so close together that you'll be frustrated if you don't see a great change. Here's a look at the four major barometers you can use to see just how effectively the Abs Diet will work for you. But for a complete picture, do all of them. Many of the standards are misleading, so your best assessment is a complete one.

• **Weight.** The heavier you are, the more at risk you are for disease and the less fit you are. While it helps gauge how well you're progressing on your diet, it doesn't take into account the amount of muscle you're going to develop. Muscle weighs about 20 percent more than fat, so even a dramatic fat loss may not translate into a dramatic drop in body weight especially at first.

• **Body mass index (BMI).** The BMI is a formula that takes into consideration your height and your weight and gives you an indication of whether you're overweight, obese, or in good shape. To calculate your BMI, multiply your weight in pounds by 703, and divide the number by your height in inches squared. For example, let's say you are 6 feet tall (that's 72 inches) and weigh 200 pounds. So first we multiply your weight by 703.

200 × 703 = 140,600

Next, we calculate your height in inches squared, meaning we multiply the number by itself.

72 × 72 = 5,184

Now we divide the first number by the second.

140,600 ÷ 5,184 = 27.1

A BMI between 25 and 30 indicates you're overweight. Over 30 signifies obesity. This measurement, too, has flaws. It doesn't take into account muscle mass, and it also leaves out another important factor—weight distribution, that is, where most of the fat on your body resides. But BMI can give you a pretty good idea of how serious your weight problem is.

back pain and Achilles tendonitis) during a year of field training. The subjects who cranked out the most situps (73 in 2 minutes) were five times less likely to suffer lower-body injuries than those who barely notched 50. But that's not all. Those who performed well in the pushups and 2-mile run enjoyed no such protection—suggesting that upper-body strength and cardiovascular endurance had little effect on injury prevention. It was abdominal strength that did it. Unlike any other muscles in your body, a strong core affects the functioning of the entire body. Think of your midsection as your body's infra-

• **Waist-to-hip ratio.** Researchers have begun using waist size and its relationship to hip size as a more definitive way to determine your health risk. This is considered more important than BMI because it measures the amount of visceral fat—the dangerous kind of fat that pushes your waist out in front of you and most threatens your organs. Because abdominal fat is the worst fat, a lower waist-to-hip ratio means fewer health risks. To figure out your waist-to-hip ratio, measure your waist at your belly button and your hips at the widest point (around your butt). Divide your waist by your hips. For example, if your hips measure 40 inches and your waist at belly button level measures 38 inches, your waist-to-hip ratio is 0.95.

38 ÷ 40 = 0.95

You want a waist-to-hip ratio of 0.92 or lower. If you were to lose just 2 inches off your waist—something you can do in just 2 weeks with the Abs Diet—you'd find yourself in the fit range.

36 ÷ 40 = 0.90

• **Body fat percentage.** Though this is the most difficult for the average person to measure because it requires a bit of technology, it's the most useful in terms of gauging how well your diet plan is working. That's because it takes into consideration not just weight but how much of your weight is fat. Many gyms offer body fat measurements through such methods as body fat scales or calipers that measure the folds of fat at several points on your body. See your local gym for what options they offer. Or try an at-home body fat calculator. I like the Tanita BC-533 Innerscan Body Composition Monitor ($120) because it measures your body's water and fat percentage as well as muscle mass, visceral fat (fat around your waist), and bone mass. If you want a simple low-tech test (and this isn't as accurate as the measurements the electronic versions will give you), try this simple exercise: Sit in a chair with your knees bent and your feet flat on the floor. Using your thumb and index finger, gently pinch the skin on top of your right thigh. Measure the thickness of the pinched skin with a ruler. If it's ¾ inch or less, you have about 14 percent body fat—ideal for a guy, quite fit for a woman. It it's 1 inch, you're probably closer to 18 percent fat, which is a tad high for a man but desirable for a woman. If you pinch more than an inch, you could be at increased risk for diabetes and heart disease. As you see your body fat percentage decrease, you'll see an increase in the amount of visible muscle. Experts say that in order for your abs to show, your body fat needs to be between 8 and 12 percent. For the average slightly overweight man, that means cutting body fat by about half.

structure. You don't want a core made of dry, brittle wood or straw. You want one made of solid steel, one that will give you a layer of protection that belly fat never could. And that's what abdominal exercises help do—build that foundation of steel.

Abs prevent back pain. Most back pain is related to weak muscles in your trunk, so maintaining a strong midsection can help resolve many back issues. The muscles that crisscross your midsection don't function in isolation; they weave through your torso like a spider web, even attaching to your spine. When your abdominal muscles are weak, the muscles in your butt (your glutes) and along the backs of your legs (your hamstrings) have to compensate for the work your abs should be doing. The effect is that core weakness destabilizes the spine and eventually leads to back pain and strain—or even more serious back problems. As you'll see in the next chapter, this program provides exercises that work your entire core—your abdominal muscles—from many different angles, so that you can develop a strong and balanced midsection.

Abs help you excel. If you play golf, basketball, tennis, or any sport that requires movement, the essential muscle group isn't your chest, biceps, or legs. It's your core. Developing core strength gives you power. It fortifies the muscles around your whole midsection and trains them to provide the right amount of support when you need it. So if you're weak off the tee, strong abs will improve your distance. If you also play stop-and-start sports like tennis or basketball, abs can improve your game tremendously by helping you get from point A to point B faster than your opponent. In essence, your legs don't control speed; your abs do. When researchers studied which muscles were the first to engage in these types of sports movements, they found that the abs fired first. The stronger they are, the faster you'll get to the ball.

THE PLAN: Work your abdominals in a circuit routine two or three times a week. I recommend that you do them before your strength-training workouts.

B = Big Muscle Groups

Muscles are what allow grooms to carry brides, football players to make tackles, and moms to carry three children, a bag of groceries, a cell phone, and car keys in one hand. But while lean muscle mass allows you to function every day and helps give your body a strong appearance and shape, muscles are also your body's oven—they broil fat at high heat. How does it work? Your muscles feed like little piranhas. They need to scour the body for calories in order to keep themselves well-nourished and growing, so they end up

"OFF CAME THE INCHES"

Name: Brandee Bratton

Age: 31

Height: 5'1"

Starting weight: 113

Six weeks later: 106

For Brandee Bratton, it was the perfect team approach: She would plan the food and meals and her husband would plan the workouts. What started out as a diet actually became more of a hobby, as the two made the program something they could do together. Starting at 113 pounds, Bratton didn't need to lose a lot of weight, but she still wanted something out of the Abs Diet.

"It's one thing to be petite, another to be strong, fit, healthy, and petite," she says.

So Bratton and her husband jumped on the program (he lost 10 pounds in 6 weeks), and Bratton wound up as a top-10 finalist in the initial Abs Diet Challenge—based largely on the way she transformed the shape of her body.

"For the first 2 weeks, I didn't notice much of a change in terms of weight. What started changing was the inches, and then the pounds just came off at the end—mostly in the thighs and hips area," says Bratton, who also dropped from about 18 percent body fat to 12. "And that was when I really got excited."

Bratton, who enjoyed the interval training and healthy eating, says that the Abs Diet is one that anyone can follow because you're always satisfied.

"This diet isn't a fad diet; it follows all the scientific rules in terms of what to eat and how to eat," she says. "I can say that there's no food deprivation you feel through this. By eating six times a day, you feel satisfied. When it's time to eat, your body gets used to eating at that time, and your body lets you know—almost like it's talking to you, 'Hey, it's been 2 hours, give me something to eat.'"

Now, Bratton, who feels healthier and stronger and likes the new toned look of her body, is studying to become a personal trainer.

"Women often look for solutions through pills, milk in a can, and gadgets," she says. "I advise this program for any woman to invest in her body."

ABS FACT

8–12

Percentage of body fat
that a man needs in
order to see his abs

churning and burning the calories you're ingesting. So by adding a little more muscle mass to your body, you'll burn more calories throughout the day. In fact, each pound of muscle you have uses up to 50 calories a day just to maintain itself. So if you add just 3 pounds of muscle, you'll burn up to an extra 150 calories a day. That may not seem like much, but at that rate, you'd burn off 15 pounds of fat in a year—simply by doing *nothing*!

This program focuses on working your big muscle groups— your legs, chest, back, and shoulders—because that's where you can build the most muscle in the least amount of time. Plus, when you work your larger muscles, you fire up your metabolism by creating a longer calorie afterburn—meaning that you'll burn calories until the next time that you do a strength-training workout.

But, hey, I'm not interested in turning you into the size of a Hummer, or even an H3. I think most of us want to be lean and strong, but still muscular and toned. A Porsche of a body, perhaps? So this plan isn't about spending as much time in the gym as you spend at your keyboard. It's about spending enough time to build a solid base of lean muscle mass—enough to change your shape and enough to build some muscle that will burn fat by itself. So that's why you'll be using two primary strength-training principles that maximize muscle growth and fat-burning and minimize the time you spend exercising.

Circuit training. It's a simple program: Perform different exercises one right after another with no more than 30 seconds of rest (1 minute in some cases). For example, you'll do a set of leg exercises followed immediately by a set of an upper-body exercise, until you do a number of different exercises in a row (some programs will contain 8 to 10 different exercises; some only 4 or 5). There are two reasons circuit training works. First, by keeping you moving and cutting down the rest periods between exercises, circuit training keeps your heart rate elevated throughout your training session, maximizing your fat burn and providing tremendous cardiovascular fitness benefits. Second, circuit training keeps your workout short—you won't waste time resting between sets of an exercise.

Compound exercises. These are the exercises that call into play multiple muscle groups rather than just one. For example, with the Abs Diet workouts, I don't want you to exercise your chest on Monday and then your shoulders on Tuesday, your triceps Wednesday, and so on, the way some programs recommend. I want you to hit many different muscles at the same time and within one circuit. One study showed that you can put on 6 pounds of muscle and lose 15 pounds of fat in 6 weeks (6 weeks!) by following an exercise program that employs the compound exercises found in the Abs Diet workout. Not only do compound exercises make your workouts more fun and more challenging, but they will also increase the demands on your muscles—even though you're not actually doing more work. For instance, the squat hits a whopping 256 muscles with just one movement. These big-muscle exercises are what will lead to big-time calorie burns.

THE PLAN: Do a strength-training circuit three times a week, focusing on compound exercises that work many muscle groups.

S = Speed Work

Your body reacts to cardiovascular exercise the way you react to music. If you hear a long, slow piece of music, you'll get lulled into zone-out mode. But if you hear something that's high-energy, you can't help but jump, bob, and mosh. Sure, there are some wonderful benefits to long, slow music—anybody who's ever brought Marvin Gaye along on a date will testify to that—but your body reacts better in terms of fat loss when you engage in cardiovascular exercise that's high-energy and high-intensity. That is, the most effective cardiovascular workouts are ones that mix periods of high intensity (going close to all out) with periods of low intensity (think light jog). Bottom line: You want a Ludacris workout, not a Chopin one.

Time and time again, research has shown that higher-intensity workouts promote weight loss better than steady-state activities like running 3 or 4 miles at the same pace (Bo-o-oring!). In a Canadian study from Laval University, researchers measured differences in fat loss between two groups of exercisers following two different workout programs. The first group rode stationary bikes four or five times a week and burned 300 to 400 calories per 30- to 45-minute session. The second group did the same, but only one or two times a week, and they filled the rest of their sessions with short intervals of high-intensity cycling. They hopped on their stationary bikes and pedaled as quickly as they could for 30 to 90 seconds, rested, and then repeated the process several times per exercise session. As a result, they burned 225 to 250 calories while cycling, but they had burned more fat at the end of the study than the workers in the first group. In fact, even

A RUNNING DEBATE

The cardiovascular-exercise camp squares off against the metal heads

You're used to seeing people sweat on machines, sign up for marathons, and cycle across Iowa as a means to getting in better shape. It's true: Cardiovascular exercise—steady-state endurance exercises, like running, biking, and swimming—burns a lot of calories. In fact, it often burns more than other forms of exercise like strength training or soul-soothing workouts like yoga. And cardio helps control stress, improves your cardiovascular fitness, lowers blood pressure, and improves your cholesterol profile. I run all the time.

But when it comes to weight control, aerobic exercise builds little (if any) muscle—and muscle is the key component of a speedy metabolism. Here's the problem with low-intensity aerobic exercise: Just like a car can't run without gas or a kite can't fly without wind, a body can't function without food. Generally, during exercise, your body calls upon glycogen (the stored form of carbohydrate in muscles and the liver), fat, and, in some cases, protein. When you're doing low-intensity aerobic exercise like jogging, your body primarily uses fat and glycogen (carbohydrates) for fuel. When it continues at longer periods (20 minutes or more), your body drifts into depletion: You exhaust your first-tier energy sources (your glycogen stores), and your body hunts around for the easiest source of energy it can find—protein. Well, guess what your muscles are made of? To feed itself during a long aerobic workout, your body actually begins to eat up muscle tissue, converting the protein stored in your muscles into the energy you need to keep going. Once your body reaches that plateau, it burns up 5 to 6 grams of protein for every 30 minutes of ongoing exercise. By burning protein, you're not only missing an opportunity to burn fat but also losing all-important and powerful muscle. So aerobic exercise actually decreases muscle mass. Decreased muscle mass ultimately slows down your metabolism, making it easier for you to gain weight.

Now here's an even more shocking fact: When early studies compared cardiovascular exercise to weight training, researchers learned that those who engaged in aerobic activities burned more calories during exercise than those who weight trained. You'd assume, then, that aerobic exercise was the way to go. But that's not the end of the story.

It turns out that while lifters didn't burn as many calories during their workouts as the folks who ran or biked, they burned far more calories over the course of the next several hours. This phenomenon is known as the afterburn—the additional calories your body burns off in the hours and days after a workout. When researchers looked at the metabolic increases after exercise, they found that the increased metabolic effect of aerobics lasted only 30 to 60 minutes. The effects of weight training lasted as long as 48 hours. That's 48 hours during which the body was burning additional fat.

though they exercised less, their fat loss was nine times greater. Researchers said that the majority of the fat burning took place after the workout. (See "A Running Debate," opposite, for more on steady-state cardiovascular exercise.) And that's really what makes it so effective—you'll keep your fat-burning mechanisms revved not only *during* your exercise but *after* it as well.

THE PLAN: Do one 20-minute interval workout per week to complement your strength training. Pick a traditional cardiovascular exercise (running, swimming, biking, cardiovascular machine), and alternate between periods of high intensity and periods of lower intensity. On your off days, I'd encourage you to do 30 minutes of brisk walking or a light workout with the cardiovascular exercise of your choice—as a way to increase your weekly calorie burn. As you advance, you can add another weekly interval workout.

ABS FACT

2

Percentage of women with a model's body

3 = 3 Times per Week

Go back to the study where subjects added 6 pounds of muscle and lost 15 pounds of fat using compound exercises. Their workout? They followed an exercise plan for only 20 minutes three times a week. That's it. In order to make this work, that's all the time you need. Of course, you can spend more time if you want—and as you get stronger. You'll maximize your fat burn by adding one other interval workout to your schedule, for instance, and you'll also see a speedier weight loss by doing something light—like brisk walking—on your off days. And if you're like the many other people who have succeeded on the Abs Diet, you'll find that exercise is a little bit like a bag of potato chips—once you've dug in, you won't want to stop. Once you start seeing results, you'll push to accelerate them even more. But you have to be careful, because exercise is like a bag of chips in another way, too: You can OD on it, which will negate all the gains you've made. For instance, you don't want to strength train any more than three times a week (your muscles grow when they're at rest). Plus, by keeping your workout schedule balanced throughout the week, you'll achieve one of the main goals you should have with any exercise program: Finish one workout looking forward to—not dreading—your next one.

ABS DIET SUCCESS STORY

"FINALLY HAPPY ABOUT MY SHAPE"

Name: Mike Mendoza

Age: 30

Height: 5'8"

Starting weight: 185

Six weeks later: 167

Current weight: 156

Starting waist size: 37"

Current waist size: 30"

Mike Mendoza struggled all his life with weight issues. He wasn't extremely overweight, but he was always the kid who was 15 or 20 pounds heavier than the rest of them.

"I always knew I carried a little extra, but people figure that's just your build. My wife would always say, 'That's just the way you're built,'" he says. "But I was flabby and I was hoping to eliminate fat in the chest area. That was really embarrassing growing up, not wanting to take my shirt off."

Mendoza used to lift really hard—up to 2 hours a day. But all he did was put on muscle *under* the fat because he wasn't watching his diet. So he was never really able to get lean.

When he read about the Abs Diet, he decided to try it because it gave him the ability to eat six meals a day—and still have things like bread and sandwiches. Ever since, he's stuck to it. He's found the recipes he really likes and stuck to them.

Now, he does the circuit routine, and he says it's helped him add muscle, because it keeps him moving through a workout. "You hit all the body parts at one time, and it works because you keep working all the different muscle groups. I love the circuit routine."

Mendoza says the key to his success is his preparation. Every Sunday, he makes smoothies and chili and packs bags of almonds—so he's well-organized and it's easy to eat right throughout the week.

He says the Abs Diet has helped identify his bad eating habits, and he realized he didn't have to make every meal a Thanksgiving dinner in order to get enjoyment out of food. He was eating for the wrong reasons—because he was tense or stressed.

"I've learned a lot about myself," he says. "I've finally been able to be happy with the shape I'm in and steer my energy into other areas of my life and not worry about how I look. And that's just been one of the great things that's come of this."

Putting It All Together

I have the same goal with ABS3 as yogis do with Downward Dog—maximum flexibility. I want you to be able to make choices under the framework of the ABS3 guidelines—to be able to adapt workouts based on your own life. When you construct your schedule, make sure to:

- Leave at least 48 hours between weight workouts. Your muscles need time to recover and repair themselves after a workout. Walk or go for a light run instead.

- Take 1 day each week to rest, with no formal exercise.

- Before starting to exercise, warm up for 5 minutes, either through a light jog, riding on a stationary bike, jumping rope, or doing slow jumping jacks.

- On off days, you can do optional cardiovascular exercise, such as cycling, swimming, or running. Light cardiovascular exercise like brisk walking is recommended for 2 of your 3 days off.

ABS FACT

20

Percentage drop in heart-disease risk by burning 1,000 to 2,500 calories a week exercising

The three components of your weekly schedule include:

A = Abdominal Exercises

Twice a week. I recommend doing them before your strength training or interval workouts.

B= Big Muscle Groups

Strength training three times a week. These are total-body workouts, with one workout that puts extra emphasis on your legs.

(S) = Speed Intervals

Once a week.

For suggested weekly schedules, see the next page.

THE ABS DIET
SUGGESTED WEEKLY
SCHEDULES

THIS AT-A-GLANCE GUIDE gives you suggested options for planning your training programs.

IF YOU HAVE TIME FOR 3X/WEEK . . .

Monday:	Abdominal workout (10 minutes)
	Strength-training circuit (20 minutes)
Tuesday:	Off, or brisk walking for 30 minutes
Wednesday:	Strength-training circuit (20 minutes)
	Interval training (20 minutes)
Thursday:	Off, or brisk walking for 30 minutes
Friday:	Abdominal workout (10 minutes)
	Strength-training circuit (20 minutes)
Saturday:	Off, or brisk walking for 30 minutes
Sunday:	Brisk walking for 1 hour

IF YOU HAVE TIME FOR 4X/WEEK . . .

Monday:	Abdominal workout (10 minutes)
	Strength-training circuit (20 minutes)
Tuesday:	Off, or brisk walking for 30 minutes
Wednesday:	Strength-training circuit (20 minutes)
Thursday:	Interval training (20–30 minutes)
Friday:	Abdominal workout (10 minutes)
	Strength-training circuit (20 minutes)
Saturday:	Off, or brisk walking for 30 minutes
Sunday:	Brisk walking for 1 hour

IF YOU HAVE TIME FOR 5X/WEEK . . .

Monday:	Abdominal workout (10 minutes)
	Strength-training circuit (20 minutes)
Tuesday:	Interval training (20–30 minutes)
Wednesday:	Strength-training circuit (20 minutes)
Thursday:	Interval training (20–30 minutes)
Friday:	Abdominal workout (10 minutes)
	Strength-training circuit (20 minutes)
Saturday:	Off, or brisk walking for 30 minutes
Sunday:	Brisk walking for 1 hour

IF YOU HAVE TIME FOR 6X/WEEK . . .

Monday:	Abdominal workout (10 minutes)
	Strength-training circuit (20 minutes)
Tuesday:	Interval training (20–30 minutes)
Wednesday:	Strength-training circuit (20 minutes)
Thursday:	Interval training (20–30 minutes)
Friday:	Abdominal workout (10 minutes)
	Strength-training circuit (20 minutes)
Saturday:	Fun day: Recreational sport/time of your choice
Sunday:	Take a day off, would ya?

Chapter 2

ABS3: ABDOMINAL EXERCISES

Build a Strong Core by Working Your Abdominals and Lower Back

AS I SAID IN THE PREVIOUS CHAPTER, abdominal exercises themselves will not burn fat, but you want to strengthen your abs so they're there to show off for when the fat does vanish. Build a strong core and your abdominals will pop out of your midsection the way Tara Reid pops out of a dress.

In the original Abs Diet book, I outlined 50-"6-pack" exercises that you could pick from—focusing on five different parts of your core region. I've included them here so that this can serve as the ultimate abdominal reference manual, and I've also included new exercises. The first group of abdominal exercises are total-core moves that work multiple parts of your abdominals. To do that circuit, pick any five from the group and follow the instructions for The New Abs Diet Abdominals Workout as outlined on page 18 (one exercise immediately followed by another). I've also included more advanced exercises if you are already well on your way to stop-traffic abs.

But the best part about these abdominal exercises is that you can treat them like a good wardrobe—mix and match them, change them from workout to workout, try ones you've never tried before, and construct your own circuit from any of the exercises in this chapter. All you have to do is follow these guidelines:

Work your abs 2 or 3 days a week. Abs develop when they're at rest, not when you're working them. So working them every day doesn't give them a chance to grow and get strong. You will develop abs by working them two or three times a week. I'd recom-

---

ABS DIET SUCCESS STORY

"IF THERE'S A WAY, I'LL FIGURE IT OUT"

Name: Larry Redden

Age: 66

Height: 5'8"

Starting weight: 185

Six weeks later: 170

As a captain in the San Diego fire department, Larry Redden has sustained his share of injuries. He's torn his rotator cuff, injured his shoulder after taking an 8-foot fall, torn a biceps muscle, and injured his ankle. "All these things happen when you fight wildland and structure fires over the years," he says. None of the injuries happened until after he turned 50, and since then, he's had four surgeries on his left shoulder alone. "I'm not the kind that wants to sit back and mope over injuries, but I had about 3 years where I couldn't work out because my shoulder was killing me," he says.

Redden read about the Abs Diet and decided it was time to take off the extra weight he had gained from the inactivity.

"If you want a change, you've got to make a change," he says.

So Redden took to the diet and performed the weights workout at home—making adjustments and substitutions for exercises he couldn't do because of his shoulder.

"There's always another way you can work your muscle. If there's a way, I'll figure it out," he says.

"The diet really motivated me again," he says. "Basically, it gave me the control over my life I felt like I had lost as a consequence of my injuries. I felt like I didn't have control because I couldn't do the things I wanted to do. I was pretty down about that. When you're one way all your life and can't do something, you get down and feel really bad. Now I feel great. Just because you're injured doesn't mean you have to lay around on your duff and mope about it."

mend adding the ab circuit to the beginning of your strength-training workout. Saving them until the end of the workout means there's more possibility that you'll skimp and take shortcuts.

Hit the whole region. There are five regions of your abdominals that you're going to work (see page 34 for specifics). In your abs circuit, you're going to hit all areas of your abdominal muscles to ensure a complete core workout.

Pick different exercises every workout. There are hundreds of ways to work your abs, but you need to pick only five exercises each workout. The key is variety: Changing your routine doesn't allow your abs to get comfortable, so they'll continue to grow after each workout.

Do a circuit. In the first week of workouts, do just one set of each of your five exercises. (A set is 10 to 15 repetitions, depending on the exercise.) In the second and third week, do two sets if you'd like, but perform them in circuits—that is, do all of the exercises once before repeating any of them. After that, you can increase to three circuits. Even then, your ab workouts shouldn't take more than 10 minutes.

Go slow. Each rep of an ab exercise should last slightly longer than Richard Hatch's fame—4 to 6 seconds. Any faster, and you run the risk of letting momentum do the work. The slower you go, the higher the intensity. The higher the intensity, the stronger the stomach.

The New Abs Diet Abdominals Workout

How to Do It: Pick any five exercises from this list and perform in a circuit with no more than 30 seconds of rest (1 minute in some cases)—one exercise followed by the next. Rest. After Week 1, repeat the circuit. Some exercises use such equipment as medicine balls, dumbbells, or cable machines—and with some of the more advanced moves, you'll need a partner. If you're just starting out, pick beginner exercises. As you progress, experiment with different exercises (using a smaller number of repetitions or eliminating equipment) to get the feel of more advanced moves.

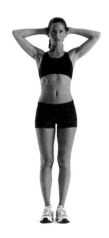
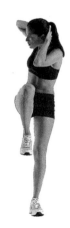

STEAM ENGINE

Stand with your hands behind your head. Touch your left elbow to your right knee by bending and raising the knee while crunching your left armpit toward your right hip. Return to the starting position and repeat to the opposite side, crunching your right armpit toward your left hip.

16–20 repetitions [*Beginner*]

"THANKS, ABS DIET!"

JOSH HANSEN

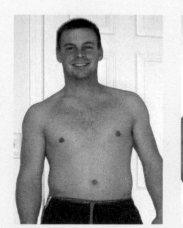
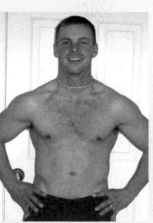

WEIGHT, WEEK 1: 183
WEIGHT, WEEK 6: 162

"I've been struggling with the reality I'm closer to 30 now than 20, though my body knew this long ago. A new dad, I had no energy and spent any free time napping. I desperately needed a change, but I lacked motivation. My wife bought me both Abs books and I went from fries to spinach, almonds, and turkey; and now I'm actually reading food labels. I'm lifting weights again and cooking for the whole family. This isn't a diet, it's a lifestyle!"

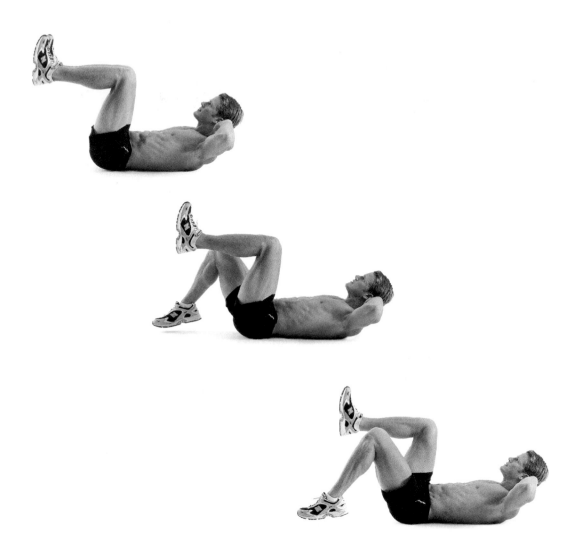

TOE TAP

Lie on your back and place your hands behind your ears. Lift your legs until your knees are above your hips and your lower legs are parallel to the floor. Press your lower back against the floor and crunch forward until your shoulders are off the floor. With your toes pointed down, lower your right foot as far as you can without lifting your back off the floor. Return to the starting position and repeat with your left leg.

10 repetitions [*Beginner to intermediate*]

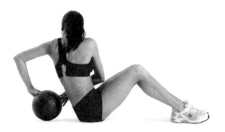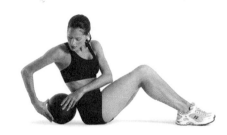

SEATED TWIST

Sit on the floor, your back straight but leaning slightly toward the floor, as if in the "up" position of a situp. Your knees should be bent 90 degrees, your feet about 15 inches apart and resting on the floor. (Your feet can either stay flat or you can raise your toes so that just your heels are touching the floor.) Hold a medicine ball close to your chest, rotate your torso to the left, and place the ball on the floor behind you. Rotate around to the right, pick up the ball, rotate left, and place it behind you.

16–20 repetitions [*Intermediate*]

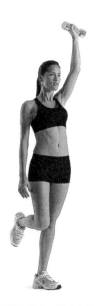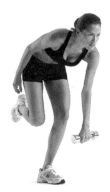

SINGLE-LEG WOOD CHOP

Hold a light dumbbell in your left hand with a straight arm, above your shoulder. Bend your right knee 90 degrees to lift your right foot behind you. Balancing on your left leg, forcefully swing the dumbbell down toward your right hip. (Don't move it behind you.) Then bring it back to the starting position. Do half the repetitions, then switch sides.

16–20 repetitions [*Intermediate*]

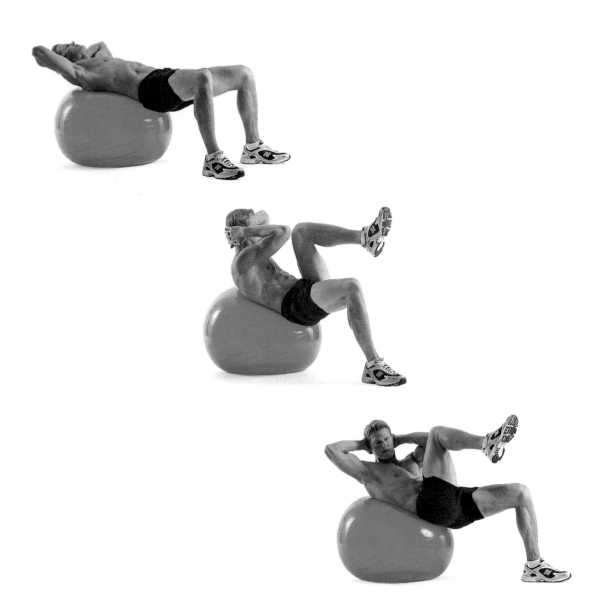

BALL BICYCLE

Lie on your back on a stability ball with your knees bent at 90 degrees, your feet flat, and your hands behind your ears. Keeping your right foot planted, lift your left foot off the floor and bring your left knee to meet your right elbow. Do half the repetitions, then switch legs.

16–20 repetitions [*Intermediate*]

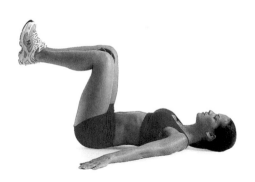
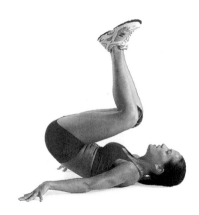
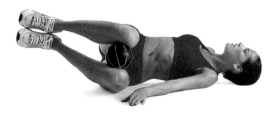
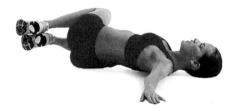

REVERSE CRUNCH WITH KNEE DROP

Lie on your back, hands resting on the floor at your sides, hips and knees bent 90 degrees, and feet off the floor. Position a medicine ball between your knees. Keep your lower back on the floor throughout the exercise. Contract your abdominals and pull your knees to your chest, then return them to the starting position. Lower your knees to the left and return to the starting position. Drop your knees to your right on the next repetition; alternate sides for each rep.

10 repetitions [*Intermediate to advanced*]

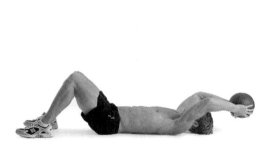
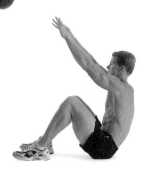

MEDICINE BALL THROW

Holding a light medicine ball in both hands, lie faceup on the floor with your back flat and your knees bent. Extend your arms beyond your head so the ball is just above the floor. Your partner sits 5 to 10 feet in front of you with his feet flat on the floor, knees bent, and arms straight overhead so he's ready to catch your pass. Keeping your arms straight, curl your body up and throw the ball to your partner's hands. Remain in the sitting position. After he catches the ball, he should throw the ball back to you. Lower yourself as you catch it.

12–15 repetitions [*Intermediate to advanced*]

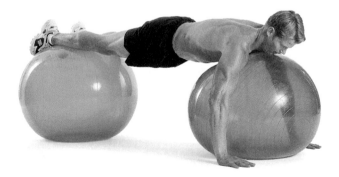

SWISS BALL STABILITY POSE

Lie facedown across two Swiss balls. Your body should be straight, with your chest lying on the first ball and your knees and shins resting on the other. With your feet spaced 12 to 18 inches apart, place your hands on the floor for balance and hold the position for 60 seconds. As you gain strength, place your hands on the side of the ball, or hold your arms out in front of you.

2 sets of 60 seconds [*Intermediate to advanced*]

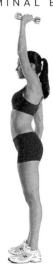
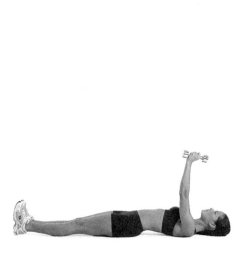

TURKISH GETUP

Lie on your back with your legs straight. Hold a dumbbell in your left hand with your arm straight above your chest. Keeping your elbow locked, move the weight above your head as you stand up. (Move your legs and right arm underneath you to push yourself up.) Still keeping your arm straight and the weight above you, reverse the steps to return to the starting position.

4 repetitions each side [*Advanced*]

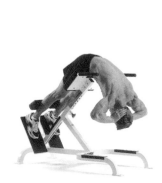
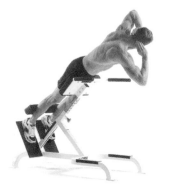
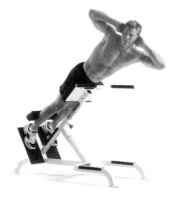

BENCH RAISE

Lie facedown on a back extension station with your torso hanging off the end. Your hips should rest along the edge of the bench so you can bend at the waist. Raise your torso until your body is perfectly straight and level, and extend your arms out to the sides. Slowly twist your torso to the left. Pause, then slowly lower yourself back down.

12–16 repetitions [*Advanced*]

ABS DIET SUCCESS STORY

"TURNING 40 WAS THE WAKEUP CALL"

Name: David Shahan

Age: 41

Height: 5'9"

Starting weight: 187

Six weeks later: 173

Starting body fat percentage: 19

Six weeks later: 9

Starting waist size: 34

Six weeks later: 31

David Shahan started the Abs Diet right after he turned 40. He'd been in shape and played sports, but building a career and family meant that he wasn't the same guy he used to be. Plus, his father had died of a heart attack and his own cholesterol numbers were climbing. "There were some vain reasons for starting, but some real health concerns, too," he says.

Shahan was drawn to the Abs Diet because he liked so many of the foods on the Power 12 list. Now he grazes all day long and doesn't worry much about quantities. "I can have a big bowl of oatmeal with walnuts in the morning and not worry about it because it's good food," he says.

To kickstart his metabolism, Shahan went to two workouts a day—interval cardio sessions in the morning and strength training at lunch. Long-term, that's hard to maintain, he says, but it helped burn fat initially. The other downside? "My wife hated the laundry it generated."

Now, he's dropped his cholesterol (from 256 to 180), firmed up, and overall feels much better about himself.

"I have a lot more energy. With two small kids, it was hard coming home from a full day of work and they're ready to jump and play. Now, it's a heckuva lot easier," Shahan says. "And your self-esteem goes up, and that confidence carries over with everything you're doing, business and personal. It's affected all aspects of my life, really. Your self-esteem and self-image have such an impact on everything you do. You don't realize it until you improve it, and it's like, Wow."

The Advanced Abs Workout

How to Do It: Pick any three or four exercises from this list and perform in a circuit with no more than 30 seconds rest (1 minute in some cases)—one exercise followed by the next. Rest, then repeat the circuit. Abdominal masochists like Matthew McConaughey can do all six in the circuit, then repeat.

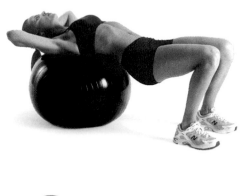

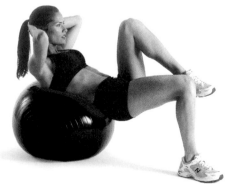

SWISS BALL CRUNCH/KNEE TUCK

Sit on top of the Swiss ball with your legs in front of you, feet flat on the floor, and hands behind your head. Keeping your feet flat on the floor, slowly lean back along the ball until your head, shoulders, and back are lying comfortably along its surface. Slowly curl and lift your shoulders and upper back up from the ball as you simultaneously draw your left knee toward your chest. Lower your left foot back down as you lower your torso down to the ball. Repeat the motion, this time raising your right knee up toward your chest as you crunch up. Keep the ball still. Lower yourself back down and repeat the exercise, alternating between your left leg and your right.

12–16 repetitions

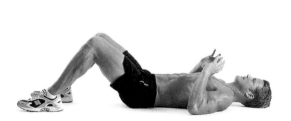

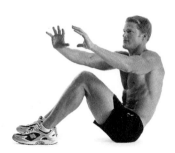

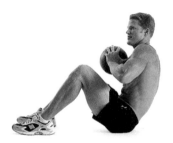

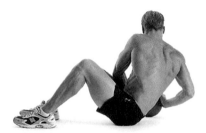

TWISTING MEDICINE BALL TOSS

Lie faceup on the floor with your hands resting next to your chest. Keep your knees bent and feet flat. Have a partner stand a few feet in front of you and to your right. Curl and lift up so that your torso is almost perpendicular to the floor and extend your arms out in front of your chest. Now, have your partner toss the ball across your body to your left side. Catch the ball with both hands and slowly twist your body to your left, lowering your torso as you go. Touch the ball to the floor as your partner moves to your left. Curl yourself up and toss the ball back to your partner. Repeat the exercise, with your partner throwing the ball across your body to your right. Catch the ball, twist to the right as you lower yourself down, and touch the ball to the floor. Continue the exercise, alternating from side to side.

12–16 repetitions

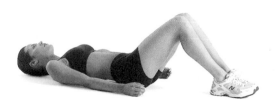

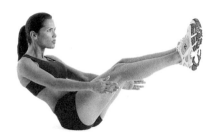

V-RAISE

Lie faceup on the floor with your hips and knees bent at 90-degree angles and your arms at your sides, palms facing in. Slowly extend your legs out and up so they are above the floor at a 45-degree angle. As you extend your legs, simultaneously raise your upper body off the floor so that your torso is held at a 45-degree angle (you should look like the letter V) and extend your arms straight out in front of you until they are parallel to the floor. Your hands should rest on the outside of your legs. Hold this position, then lower both your upper and lower body down to the floor.

12–16 repetitions

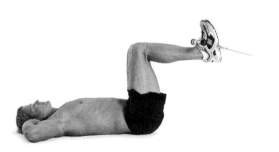 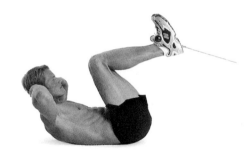

SINGLE-RESISTANCE DOUBLE CRUNCH

Place a mat in front of a low-pulley cable with a bar attached to it. Sit facing the pulley with your knees bent. Place the bar between your feet, then draw your legs together so that the chain becomes locked between your feet and the bar rests across the tops of your feet. Lean back on the mat with your head and back flat on the floor and bend your knees to a 90-degree angle (thighs perpendicular to the floor). Place your hands lightly along the sides of your head, elbows out to the sides. Holding your knees at a 90-degree angle, slowly curl your head and shoulders off the floor as you tilt your pelvis and curl your legs toward your chest. Don't draw your knees into your chest. Hold this position for 1 second, then return to the starting position (back flat on the floor with your knees bent at a 90-degree angle).

12–16 repetitions

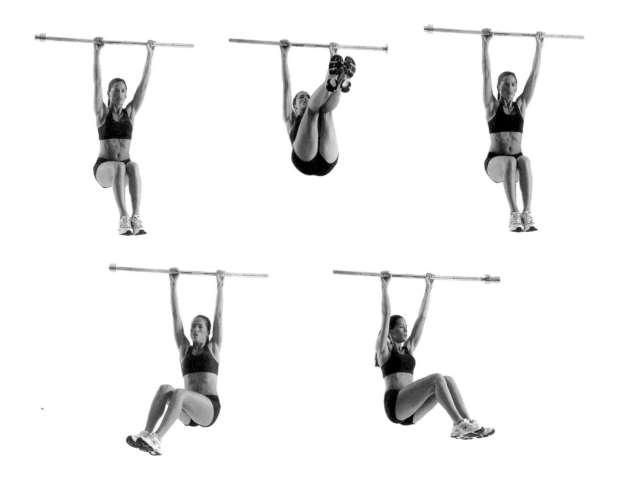

HANGING REVERSE TRUNK TWIST

Hang from a chinup bar with your hands shoulder-width apart and legs straight but bent forward at a 30-degree angle. Keeping your legs held at that angle, raise them up in front of you until your thighs are parallel to the floor. Next, tense your abs, tilt your pelvis, and slowly raise your legs up until your feet are almost as high as your head. From the side, your body will be in a V position. Don't use momentum to swing your legs up; that will engage your hip flexors, not your abdominals. Slowly lower your legs back down to the middle position, keeping your thighs parallel to the floor. Holding that posture, slowly rotate your legs to the right (as if you were pointing between 1 and 2 o'clock with your feet), then rotate your legs to the left (as if you were pointing between 10 and 11). Bring your legs back to center, slowly lower them back down, and repeat the entire cycle.

4 repetitions

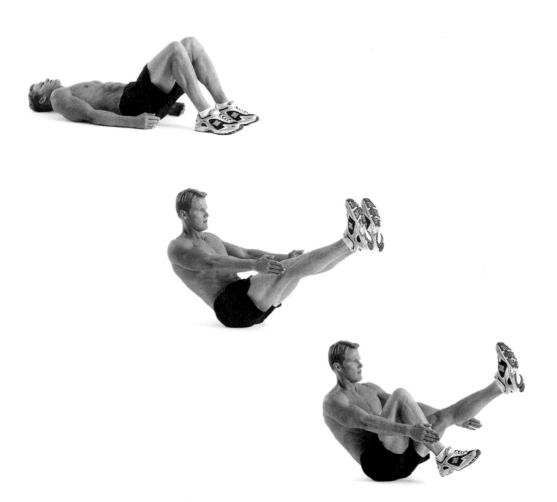

V-RAISE KNEE TUCK

Lie faceup on the floor with your hips and knees bent at 90-degree angles and your arms at your sides, palms facing in. Slowly extend your legs out and up until they are straight and 45 degrees above the floor. Simultaneously curl your shoulders and lower back off the floor, extending your hands toward the outsides of your feet so that your arms are straight out in front of you. Holding this position, slowly draw your right knee toward your chest, then extend your right leg back out. (Your left leg should remain stable throughout the movement.) Exhale as you draw your knee in and inhale as you extend your leg out. Repeat the same knee-to-chest motion with your left leg. Continue to alternate from right to left throughout the exercise.

12–16 repetitions

"I NEEDED SOMETHING THAT WAS EASY"

Name: Linda Toomey

Age: 35

Height: 5'4"

Starting weight: 145

Six weeks later: 129

When Linda Toomey had her fourth baby, she knew that she had to get the weight off. She had kept 20 pounds on from her third baby and wanted to act quickly because she knew the longer she waited, the harder it would be. Weighing 145 pounds and with four children under the age of 6, she knew that her own health—and belly—might take a back seat to everything else going on in her life. "I'm the queen of excuses," she says. She also knew that she needed as much energy as possible—especially considering she wasn't getting a full night's sleep anyway, caring for a newborn.

"At night, I expected to be tired," she says. "But I was tired 2 hours after I woke up."

Her goals: Get her body back, increase her energy, and strengthen her back to be able to meet the demands of carrying larger-than-average children.

"I tried other diets, but being so crazy and busy, I didn't have a lot of time for exercise or food preparation. I needed something that was easy and fast to prepare," Toomey says.

She found it in the Abs Diet.

"It's not really a diet," she says. "It's a lifelong eating plan. I think knowing that you can eat carbs and not resist cravings was one of the key factors. The eating plan was extremely easy to follow, and the whole family could enjoy the meals. I didn't have to prepare different foods for myself."

Toomey also included the 20-minute exercise plan and strengthened her abdominals and lower back to the point where she has no problem lifting her children.

In 6 weeks, she dropped 16 pounds and went from 36 percent body fat to 25. And she also went from a size 14 dress to size 6.

"I'm hoping it motivates a lot of women," Toomey says. "In the past after being pregnant, the waist was extremely hard for me. I may have lost inches from everywhere else in the past, but the waist was my real difficult area. It's amazing how it progressed in a short time."

The Original 50-"6-Pack" Abdominal Circuit

How to Do It: Pick one exercise from each group listed below, and do the exercise for the specified number of repetitions. Do one set of each exercise with no more than 30 seconds of rest (1 minute in some cases), and then repeat the circuit.

Note: Many of these exercises target different regions of the abdominals during the same movement, but they're grouped based on which areas they primarily work. They've also been grouped by levels of difficulty, so that you can change your workouts as you get stronger. For each exercise, pause at the end of the movement, and return to the starting position. That counts as one repetition, unless otherwise noted.

The Abs Circuit

Upper Abs: The top part of your rectus abdominis, the traditional 6-pack muscle.

Lower Abs: The lower part of the rectus abdominis.

Obliques: The muscles along the sides of your abdominal region.

Transverse Abdominis: The muscle that runs underneath your rectus abdominis, which helps give your body stability.

Lower Back: The muscles that balance your abdominal muscles and provide core strength.

UPPER ABS

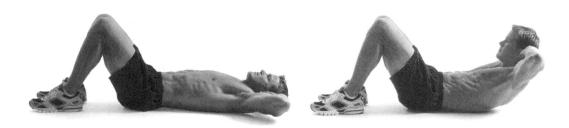

TRADITIONAL CRUNCH

Lie on your back with your knees bent and your hands behind your ears. Slowly crunch up, bringing your shoulder blades off the ground.

12–15 repetitions [*Beginner*]

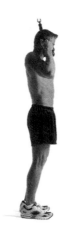 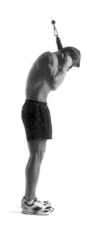

STANDING CRUNCH

Attach a rope handle to a high-cable pulley. Stand with your back to the weight stack and hold the ends of the rope on either side of your head. Crunch down.

12–15 repetitions [*Beginner*]

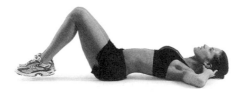 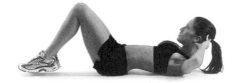

MODIFIED RAISED-FEET CRUNCH

Lie on your back with your knees bent and your hands behind your ears. Raise your feet just a few inches off the floor, and hold them there. Crunch up, then lower your torso back to the floor, keeping your feet raised throughout the movement.

12–15 repetitions [*Beginner to intermediate*]

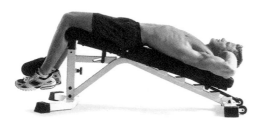 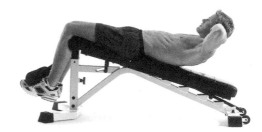

DECLINE CRUNCH

Lie on your back on a decline board, with your ankles locked under the padded support bars and your fingertips cupped behind your ears. Lift your shoulder blades off the bench, keeping your lower body flat. Don't jerk your body to build momentum. Hold the contraction for 1 second.

12–15 repetitions [*Beginner to intermediate*]

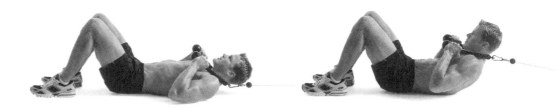

LYING CABLE CRUNCH

Attach a rope handle to the low pulley. Lie on the floor with your head near the low pulley, your knees bent, and your feet flat on the floor. Hold the handle over your chest so that the point of the rope attachment is at the base of your throat. Crunch your rib cage toward your pelvis, lifting your shoulder blades a few inches off the floor.

12–15 repetitions [*Intermediate to advanced*]

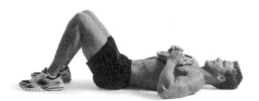 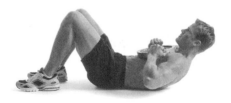

WEIGHTED CRUNCH

Lie on your back with your knees bent, holding a weight plate or dumbbell across your chest. Slowly crunch up, bringing your shoulder blades off the ground. Use progressively heavier weights.

12–15 repetitions [*Intermediate to advanced*]

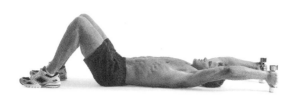 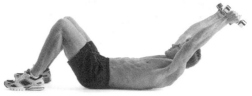

LONG-ARM WEIGHTED CRUNCH

Lie on your back with your knees bent. Hold a light dumbbell in each hand, and stretch your arms straight back behind you. Crunch your rib cage toward your pelvis. Don't generate momentum with your arms.

12–15 repetitions [*Intermediate to advanced*]

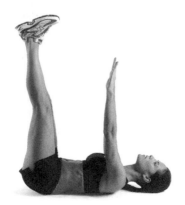 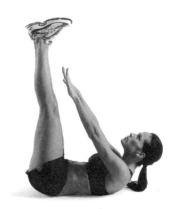

TOE TOUCH

Lie on your back with your legs raised directly over your hips; your knees should be slightly bent. Raise your arms straight up, pointing toward your toes, and relax your head and neck. Use your upper abs to raise your rib cage toward your pelvis, lift your shoulder blades off the floor, and reach toward your toes. Hold for a second. Lower your shoulders to the floor and repeat.

12–15 repetitions [*Intermediate to advanced*]

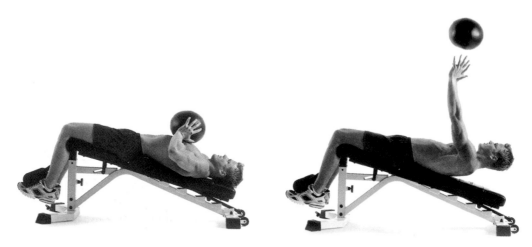

MEDICINE BALL BLAST

Set an adjustable ab bench at a 45-degree angle. Lie down on it with your head toward the floor, and hook your feet under the padded support bars. Hold a medicine ball at your chest as you lower yourself. As you come up, chest-pass the ball straight up over your head. Catch it at the top of the movement, then lower yourself and repeat.

12–15 repetitions [*Advanced*]

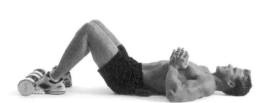

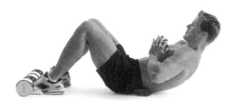

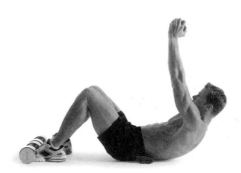

SICILIAN CRUNCH

Slide your feet under the handles of heavy dumbbells. Place a rolled-up towel under your lower back and hold a dumbbell across your chest. Raise your upper body as high as possible by crunching your rib cage toward your pelvis. At the top of the move, straighten your arms and raise the dumbbell above your head. Keep the dumbbell above your head, and take 4 seconds to lower your body to the starting position.

10 repetitions [*Advanced*]

LOWER ABS

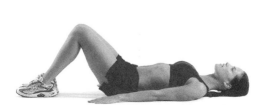 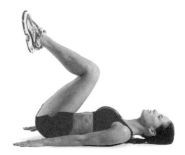

BENT-LEG KNEE RAISE

Lie on your back with your head and neck relaxed and your hands on the floor near your butt. Your knees should be bent and your feet flat on the floor. Use your lower abdominal muscles to raise your knees up toward your rib cage, then slowly lower your feet back to the starting position. As your feet lightly touch the floor, repeat.

12 repetitions [*Beginner*]

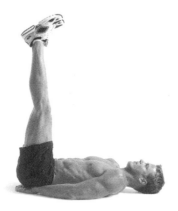 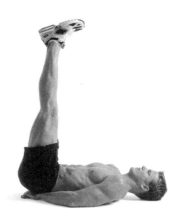

PULSE-UP

Lie with your hands underneath your tailbone and your legs raised and pointed straight up toward the ceiling, perpendicular to your torso. Pull your navel inward and flex your glutes as you lift your hips just a few inches off the floor. Then lower your hips.

12 repetitions [*Beginner*]

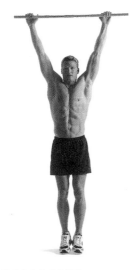
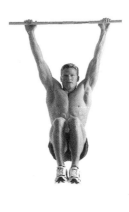

HANGING KNEE RAISE

Hang fully extended from a chinup bar, with your palms facing out and your hands a little farther than shoulder-width apart. (Your feet may lightly touch the floor.) Raise your knees toward your chest, curling your pelvis upward at the end. When you can do that for 12 repetitions, make it tougher by keeping your legs straight instead of bending your knees or by holding a medicine ball between your knees.

12 repetitions *[Beginner to intermediate]*

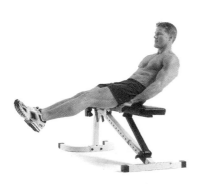
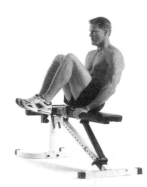

SEATED AB CRUNCH

Sit on the edge of a stable chair or bench. Place your hands in front of your butt and grip the sides of the seat. Lean back slightly and extend your legs down and away, keeping your heels 4 to 6 inches off the floor. To begin the exercise, bend your knees and slowly raise your legs toward your chest. At the same time, lean forward with your upper body, allowing your chest to approach your thighs.

12 repetitions *[Beginner to intermediate]*

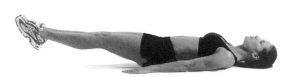
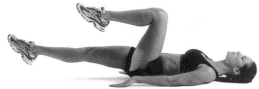

RAISED KNEE-IN

Lie on your back. Your arms should be close to your sides, with your palms down and just under your lower back and butt. Press the small of your back against the floor, and extend your legs outward, with your heels about 3 inches above the floor. Keeping your lower back against the floor, lift your left knee toward your chest. Your right leg should remain hovering above the floor. Hold, then straighten your left leg to the starting position and repeat with your right leg. Keep your abs tight throughout the exercise.

8–12 repetitions each side *[Intermediate]*

"THANKS, ABS DIET!"

DAN GALLAGHER

WEIGHT, WEEK 1: 205
WEIGHT, WEEK 6: 185

"My wakeup call came when I began taking medication for high blood pressure and lost an invincible friend to a heart attack. I hate diets because I hate feeling deprived. The abs plan is not a 'diet' but a way of life that never leaves me feeling deprived. In 6 weeks I've taken 2 inches off my waist, my blood pressure is dropping and I feel like I eat more now than I used to."

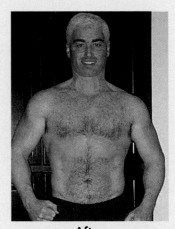

After

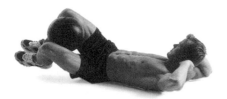

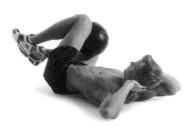

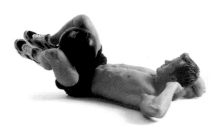

FIGURE-8 CRUNCH

Lie on your back with your knees bent at a 90-degree angle and your feet flat on the floor. Squeeze a light medicine ball tightly between your knees. Cup your hands lightly behind your ears, then slowly raise your head, shoulders, and feet off the floor. Move your knees in a wide figure-8 motion. Do 3 repetitions in one direction, then reverse the motion for 3 repetitions.

6 repetitions [*Intermediate*]

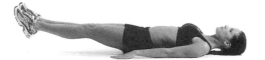

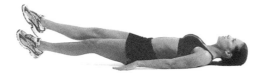

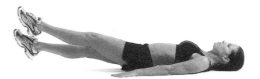

FLUTTER KICK

Lie on your back, raise both feet about a foot off the ground, and scissor-kick one leg over the other.

20 repetitions [*Intermediate*]

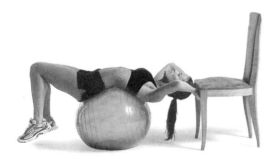
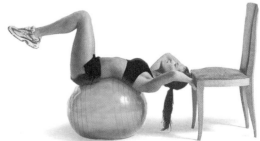

SWISS BALL KNEE RAISE

Lie faceup on a Swiss ball, with your hips lower than your shoulders. Reach back and grab something that won't move, such as a bench or a stable chair. Lift and bend your legs so that your feet are off the floor and the lower parts of your legs point ahead. (To make it more difficult, hold your legs straight out.) Do a standard Bent-Leg Knee Raise (page 40), using your abs and hip flexors to curl your knees toward your chest.

12 repetitions [*Intermediate to advanced*]

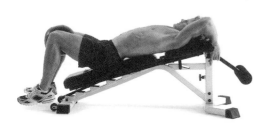
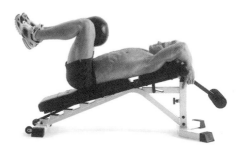

REVERSE CRUNCH HOLDING MEDICINE BALL

Lie on a slant board with your hips lower than your head. Grab the bar behind your head for support. Bend your hips and knees at 90-degree angles, and hold a small medicine ball between your knees. Start with your butt flat against the board. Pull your hips up and in toward your rib cage. Curl them as high as you can without lifting your shoulders off the board, and keep your hips and knees at 90-degree angles.

12 repetitions [*Intermediate to advanced*]

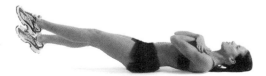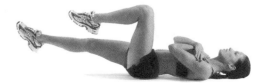

PUSH-AWAY

Lie on your back with your hands on your chest, legs extended, feet raised off the floor. Alternately bring each knee toward your head, then forcefully kick forward. Don't let your feet touch the floor. (If you feel any discomfort in your lower back while performing this exercise, try lifting your head and tucking your chin toward your chest.)

10 repetitions each side [*Intermediate to advanced*]

OBLIQUES

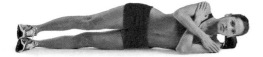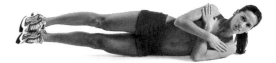

OBLIQUE V-UP

Lie on your side with your body in a straight line. Fold your arms across your chest. Keeping your legs together, lift them off the floor as you raise your top elbow toward your hip. The range of motion is short, but you should feel an intense contraction in your obliques.

10 repetitions each side [*Beginner*]

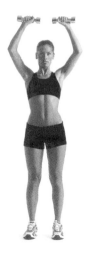

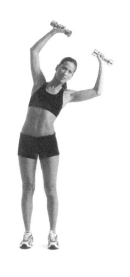

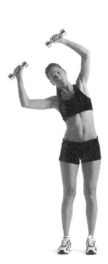

SAXON SIDE BEND

Hold a pair of lightweight dumbbells over your head, in line with your shoulders, with your elbows slightly bent. Keep your back straight, and slowly bend directly to your left side as far as possible without twisting your upper body. Pause, return to an upright position, then bend to your right side as far as possible.

6–10 repetitions on each side [*Beginner to intermediate*]

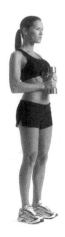
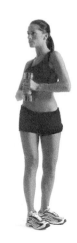

SPEED ROTATION

Stand while holding a dumbbell with both hands in front of your midsection. Twist 90 degrees to the right, then 180 degrees to your left. Keep your abs tight and move fast. Bring to center. Alternate the side you start with.

10 repetitions each side [Intermediate]

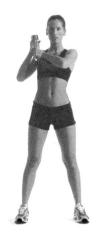
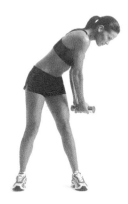

TWO-HANDED WOOD CHOP

Stand while holding a dumbbell in both hands next to your right ear. Flex your abs and rotate your torso to the left as you extend your arms and lower the dumbbell to the outside of your left knee. Lift it back, finish the set, and repeat on the other side.

10 repetitions each side [Intermediate]

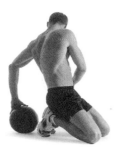
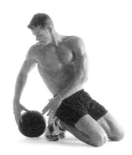

MEDICINE BALL TORSO ROTATION

Hold a medicine ball or basketball in front of you. Sit with your knees bent and your feet on the floor. Quickly twist to your left, and set the ball down behind your back. Twist to the right, and pick up the ball. Bring the ball around to your left, and set it down again. Repeat. Do the same number of repetitions in which you first twist to the left side as you do when you twist to the right side.

10 repetitions each side [Intermediate to advanced]

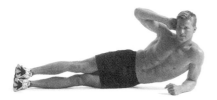
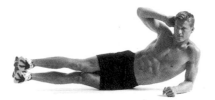

SIDE JACKKNIFE

Lie on your left side, with your legs nearly straight and slightly raised off the floor. Also raise your torso off the floor, with your left forearm on the floor for balance. Hold your other hand behind your right ear, with your elbow pointed toward your feet. Lift your legs toward your torso while keeping your torso stationary. Pause to feel the contraction on the right side of your waist. Then slowly lower your legs and repeat. Finish the set on that side, then lie on your right hip and do the same number of repetitions.

10 repetitions each side [Intermediate to advanced]

TRANSVERSE ABDOMINIS

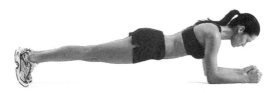

BRIDGE

Start to get in a pushup position, but bend your elbows and rest your weight on your forearms instead of on your hands. Your body should form a straight line from your shoulders to your ankles. Pull in your abdominals; imagine you're trying to move your belly button back to your spine. Hold for 20 seconds, breathing steadily. As you build endurance, you can do one 60-second set.

1–2 repetitions [*Beginner to intermediate*]

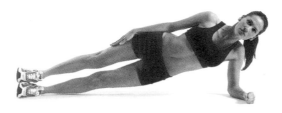

SIDE BRIDGE

Lie on your nondominant side. Support your weight with that forearm and the outside edge of that foot. Your body should form a straight line from head to ankles. Pull in your abs as far as you can, and hold this position for 10 to 30 seconds, breathing steadily. Relax. If you can do 30 seconds, do one repetition. If not, try for any combination of reps that gets you up to 30 seconds. Repeat on your other side.

1–2 repetitions on each side [*Beginner to intermediate*]

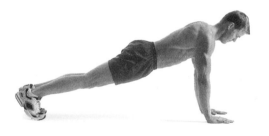

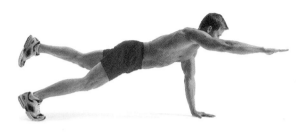

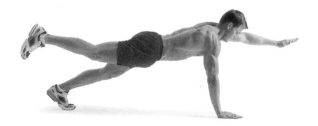

TWO-POINT BRIDGE

Get into the standard pushup position. Lift your right arm and your left leg off the floor at the same time. Hold for 3 to 5 seconds. That's one repetition. Return to the starting position, then repeat, lifting your left arm and right leg this time.

6–10 repetitions each side [Intermediate]

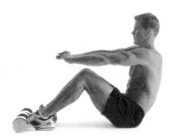
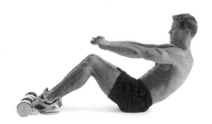

NEGATIVE CRUNCH

Sit on the floor with your knees bent and your feet flat on the floor, shoulder-width apart. Extend your arms with your fingers interlaced, palms facing your knees. Begin with your upper body at slightly less than a 90-degree angle to the floor. Lower your body toward the floor, curling your torso forward, rounding your lower back, and keeping your abs contracted. When your body reaches a 45-degree angle to the floor, return to the starting position. (*Note:* You may need to tuck your feet under a set of weights to help maintain balance throughout the exercise.)

10 repetitions [*Intermediate*]

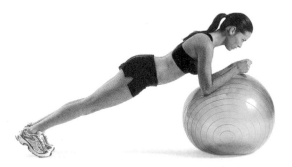

SWISS BALL BRIDGE

Rest your forearms on the ball and your toes on the floor, with your body in a straight line. Pull in your stomach, trying to bring your belly button to your spine. Hold for 20 seconds, breathing steadily. As you build endurance, you can do one 60-second set.

1–2 repetitions [*Intermediate to advanced*]

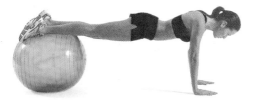 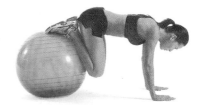

SWISS BALL PULL-IN

Get into the pushup position—your hands set slightly wider than and in line with your shoulders—but instead of placing your feet on the floor, rest your shins on a Swiss ball. With your arms straight and your back flat, your body should form a straight line from your shoulders to your ankles. Roll the Swiss ball toward your chest. Pause, then return the ball to the starting position by extending your legs to the starting position and rolling the ball backward.

5–10 repetitions [*Intermediate to advanced*]

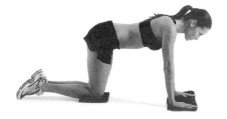 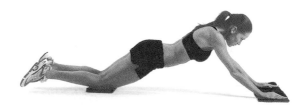

TOWEL ROLL

Kneel on a towel or mat on a tile or wooden floor. Put a towel on the floor in front of you, and place your hands on it. Slide the towel across the floor until your body is fully extended. Your body should look as if you're in a diving position. Slowly slide back up.

5–10 repetitions [*Advanced*]

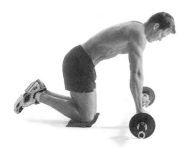
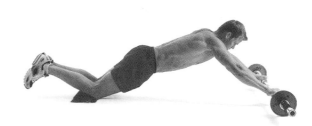

BARBELL ROLLOUT

Load a pair of 5-pound plates onto a barbell. Kneel on an exercise mat or towel, with your shoulders directly over the bar. Grab the bar with an overhand, shoulder-width grip. Start with your back in a slightly rounded position, allowing it to extend into a more neutral position as you execute the movement. Roll the bar out in front of you, holding your knees in place as your hips, torso, and arms go forward. Keeping your arms taut, advance as far as you can without arching your back or touching the floor with anything above your knees. Pause for a split second, then pull back to the starting position.

5–10 repetitions *[Advanced]*

LOWER BACK

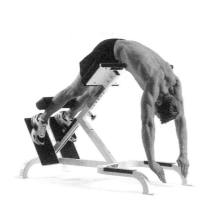
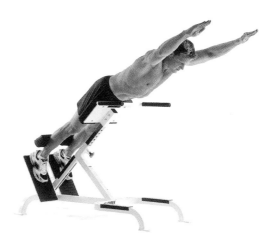

BACK EXTENSION

Position yourself in a back extension station, and hook your feet under the leg anchor. Hold your arms straight out in front of you. Your body should form a straight line from your hands to your hips. Lower your torso, allowing your lower back to round, until it's just short of perpendicular to the floor. Raise your upper body until it's slightly above parallel to the floor. At this point, you should have a slight arch in your back, and your shoulder blades should be pulled together. Pause for a second, then repeat.

12–15 repetitions *[Beginner to intermediate]*

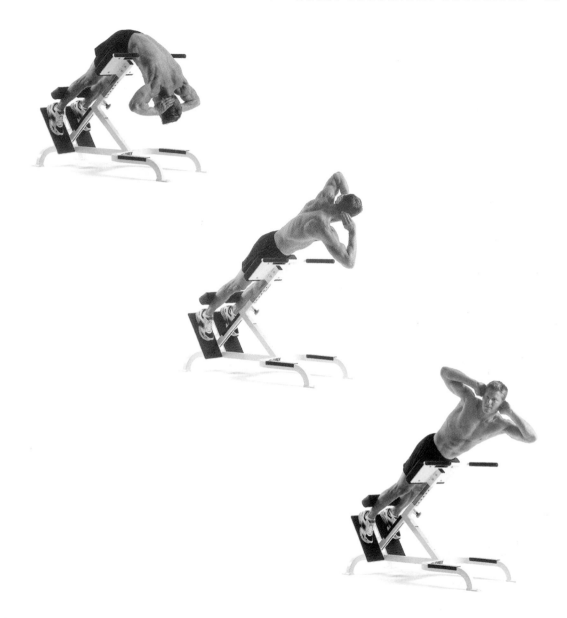

TWISTING BACK EXTENSION

Position yourself in a back extension station, and hook your feet under the leg anchor. Place your fingers lightly behind or over your ears. Lower your upper body, allowing your lower back to round, until it's just short of perpendicular to the floor. Raise and twist your upper body until it's slightly above parallel to the floor and facing left. Pause, then lower your torso and repeat, this time twisting to the right.

12–15 repetitions [*Intermediate*]

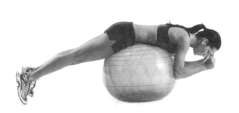 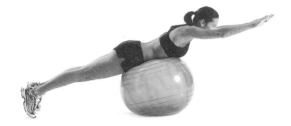

SWISS BALL SUPERMAN

Lie facedown over a Swiss ball so that your hips are pressed against the ball and your torso is rounded over it. Lift your upper arms so that they're parallel to your body, and bend your elbows 90 degrees so that your fingers are pointing forward and your elbows are pointing back. Slowly extend your back until your chest is completely off the ball, extend your arms forward, and hold that position. Draw your arms back into position as you return your torso to the ball.

12–15 repetitions [*Intermediate*]

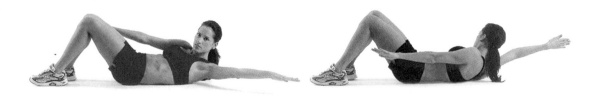

SWIMMER'S BACKSTROKE

Lie faceup on the floor, with your knees bent and feet flat. Flatten your lower back against the floor. Now do a crunch to flex your trunk forward, and lift your shoulder blades as high off the floor as you possibly can. Keeping your chest high, perform a backstroke with one arm at a time, allowing your torso to twist toward the arm that's reaching back. Work up to 5 repetitions of 45 seconds each, alternating arms. The higher you lift your chest off the floor, the better your exercise will work. Add light dumbbells when the move becomes too easy.

1–5 repetitions [*Intermediate to advanced*]

All-in-One Ab Moves

Looking to shave even more time off your workout while shaving fat from your waistline? The remaining 18 moves work several areas of your midsection simultaneously. Use any one of the following substitutions to cover two or three areas with one exercise and you can reduce your workout plan to just a few exercises instead of five.

CRUNCH/SIDE BEND COMBO

Targets both the upper abs and obliques

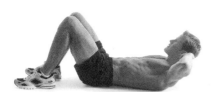 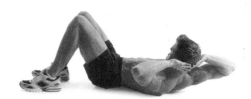

Lie on your back, with your knees bent and your hands behind your ears. Curl up so that your shoulder blades are off the floor. Bend at the waist to the left, aiming your left armpit toward your right hip. Straighten, then bend to your right.

8 repetitions to each side *[Beginner]*

"THANKS, ABS DIET!"

GEORGE SNARBERG

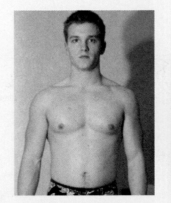 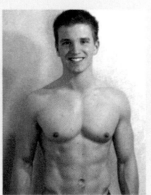

WEIGHT, WEEK 1: 175
WEIGHT, WEEK 6: 163

"Six weeks after signing up for the Abs Diet, I'm a completely different person, inside and out. Every day I wake up feeling better about myself. Two weeks ago I came home and told my mom that I'm going to be famous. The Abs Diet has given me the confidence I needed to pursue a career in modeling and acting. You'll be seeing me soon, looking back at you from the cover of *Men's Health*!"

SINGLE-KNEE CRUNCH

Targets both the upper and lower abs

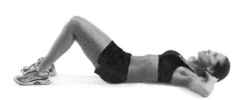 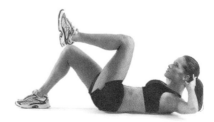

Lie on your back, with your knees bent and your feet flat on the floor. Touch the sides of your head, with your elbows bent. Raise your head, shoulders, and butt off the floor as you simultaneously bring your left knee toward your chest. Lower your torso and leg back down, then repeat the exercise, this time drawing your right knee up as you crunch.

10 repetitions each side [*Beginner to intermediate*]

TWISTING CRUNCH

Targets both the upper abs and obliques

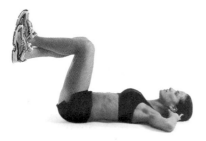 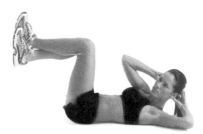

Lie on your back on the floor, with your hands cupped behind your ears and your elbows out. Cross your ankles, with your knees slightly bent, and raise your legs until your thighs are perpendicular to your body. Bring your right shoulder off the floor as you cross your right elbow over to your left knee. Return to the starting position and repeat, beginning with the left shoulder, crossing your left elbow over to your right knee.

8 repetitions to each side [*Beginner to intermediate*]

STICK CRUNCH

Targets both the upper and lower abs

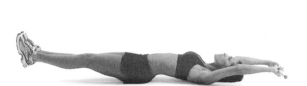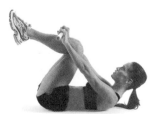

Lie on your back, with your feet raised off the ground and your knees slightly bent. Hold a broomstick in both hands behind and above your head, with your arms extended. Crunch your torso up and draw your knees up so that the stick extends past your knees. Pause, then return to the starting position.

12 repetitions *[Intermediate]*

BICYCLE

Targets both the upper and lower abs

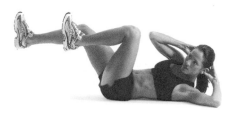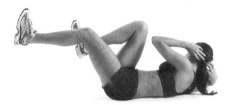

Lying on your back with your knees bent 90 degrees and your hands behind your ears, pump your legs back and forth, bicycle-style, as you rotate your torso from side to side by moving an armpit (not an elbow) toward the opposite knee.

20 repetitions *[Intermediate]*

WEIGHTED ONE-SIDED CRUNCH

Targets both the upper abs and obliques

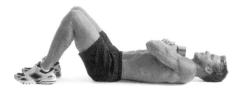 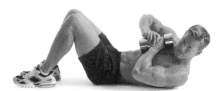

Lie with your knees bent and feet flat on the floor. Hold a dumbbell by your right shoulder with both hands. Curl your torso up and rotate to the left. Lower your upper body, finish the set, and then repeat holding the dumbbell next to your left shoulder.

8 repetitions to each side *[Intermediate]*

"THANKS, ABS DIET!"

JOHN BOYLE

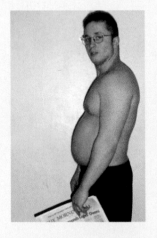 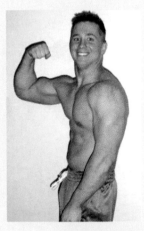

WEIGHT, WEEK 1: 194
WEIGHT, WEEK 6: 178

"I was working 60 to 70 hours a week. I felt like I had neither the time nor the motivation to brush my teeth, let alone to train and eat right. I finally realized that I was really out of shape when my girlfriend was calling me J.B., which I thought meant John Boyle, until I found out a week later it meant Jelly Belly! Right then I knew I *needed* a plan to get back in shape. With the Abs Diet, I accomplished my mission."

OBLIQUE HANGING LEG RAISE

Targets both the lower abs and obliques

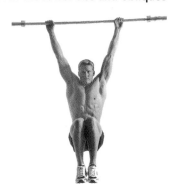

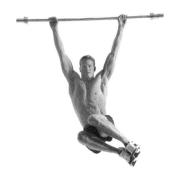

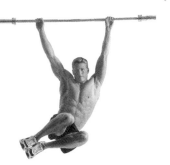

Grasp a chinup bar with an overhand grip and hang from it at arm's length, with your knees bent. Maintaining the bend in your knees, lift your left hip toward your left armpit, until your lower legs are nearly parallel to the floor. Pause, return to the starting position, and lift your right hip toward your right armpit.

10 repetitions each side [*Intermediate*]

HANGING SINGLE-KNEE RAISE

Targets both the lower abs and obliques

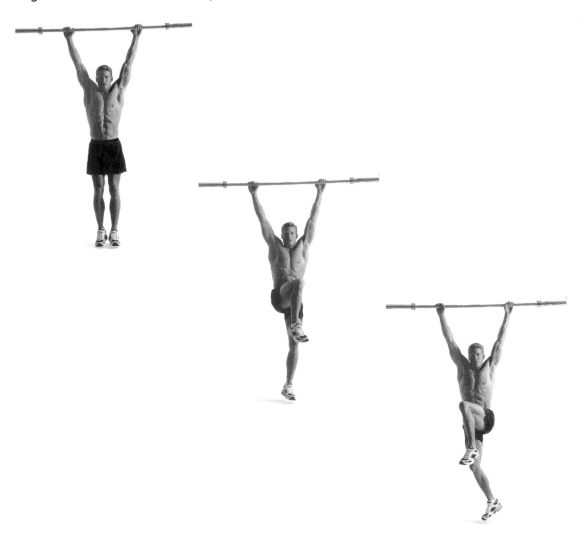

Hang fully extended from a chinup bar, with your palms facing out and your hands a little farther than shoulder-width apart. Your feet should lightly touch the floor. Without swinging to pick up momentum, raise your right knee toward your left shoulder as far as you can, using your abs for power. It's okay to tip your pelvis slightly forward to help, but don't rock. Hold for a second, then return to the starting position. Repeat with your left leg, raising it toward your right shoulder.

8–12 repetitions each side [Intermediate]

KNEELING THREE-WAY CABLE CRUNCH

Targets both the upper abs and obliques

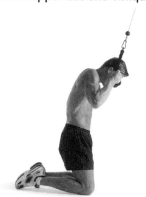 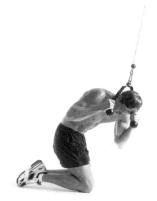

Attach a rope handle to the high pulley. Kneel facing the pulley and grab the ends of the rope, with your palms facing each other. Hold the ropes alongside your face, with your elbows bent. Bend forward at the waist, rounding your back and aiming your chest at your pelvis. Stop when you feel a contraction in your abdominal muscles. Return to the starting position, then repeat the movement, this time aiming your chest toward your left knee. Stop when you feel a contraction in your left obliques. Return, then repeat the movement to your right. That's 1 repetition.

8 repetitions [*Intermediate to advanced*]

RUSSIAN TWIST

Targets both the upper abs and obliques

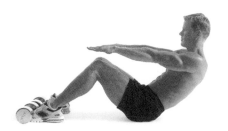 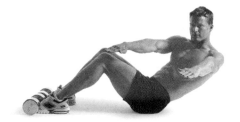

Sit on the floor, with your knees bent and your feet flat. Hold your arms straight out in front of your chest, with your palms facing down. Lean back so that your torso is at a 45-degree angle to the floor. Twist to the left as far as you can, pause, then reverse your movement and twist all the way back to the right as far as you can. As you get stronger, hold a light weight in your hands as you do the movement. (*Note:* You may need to tuck your feet under a set of weights to help maintain balance throughout the exercise.)

10 repetitions each side [*Intermediate to advanced*]

V-SPREAD TOE TOUCH

Targets both the upper abs and obliques

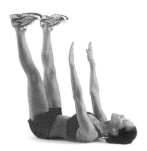

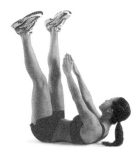

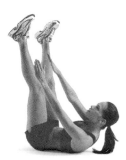

Lie flat on your back, with your legs straight up in a V position, without locking your knees. Raise your arms toward the ceiling. Curl your shoulder blades up and reach toward your right foot with both hands. Hold for a second, concentrating on your abs, then lower to the starting position. Repeat, this time reaching for your left foot. Don't pause at the starting position.

12–15 repetitions [*Intermediate to advanced*]

CORKSCREW

Targets both the lower abs and obliques

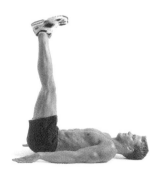 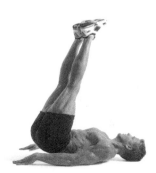

Lie on your back, with your legs raised directly over your hips; your knees should be slightly bent. Place your hands with the palms down at your sides. Use your lower abs to raise your hips off the floor and toward your rib cage, elevating your hips straight up toward the ceiling. Simultaneously twist your hips to the right in a corkscrew motion. Hold, then return to the starting position. Repeat, twisting to the left.

10 repetitions [*Intermediate to advanced*]

"THANKS, ABS DIET!"

JAMES ARRENDALE

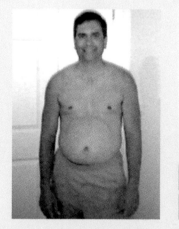 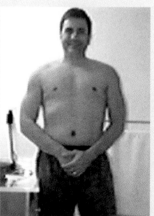

WEIGHT, WEEK 1: 197
WEIGHT, WEEK 6: 183

"From the boardroom to the bedroom, the Abs Diet made a tremendous difference in my life! Not only has my wife of 18 years started looking at me in a different way but my colleagues at work have also begun treating me with a whole new level of respect. Let's face it, from high school to the corporate world, the 'in crowd' has one thing in common: Those who fit the mold are also fit."

STRAIGHT-LEG CYCLING CRUNCH

Targets both the upper and lower abs

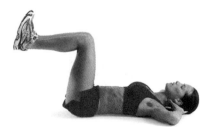

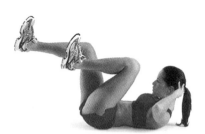

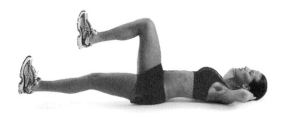

Lie on your back. Lift your legs and bend your knees 90 degrees so that your feet are in the air. Place your hands behind your ears and perform an abdominal crunch by lifting your head and shoulders off the floor. At the same time, lift your left leg to your chest. Lower your torso to the floor as you straighten your left leg, keeping it a few inches off the floor. Repeat the exercise, this time drawing your right knee up as you crunch. Alternate from left to right throughout the exercise.

10 repetitions each side [*Advanced*]

LATERAL MEDICINE BALL BLAST

Targets both the upper abs and obliques

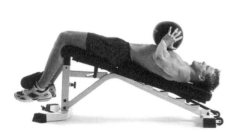 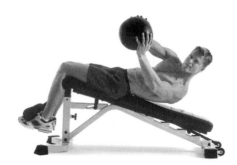

Set an adjustable ab bench at a 45-degree angle. Lie down on it, and hook your feet under the padded support bars. Hold a medicine ball or weight plate against your chest. As you come up, twist to the left and extend your arms as if you were throwing the ball or weight. Pull it back to your chest as you untwist and lower yourself. Repeat, twisting to the right.

5 repetitions each side [*Advanced*]

"THANKS, ABS DIET!"

STEPHEN GRAY

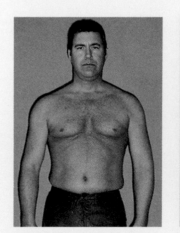 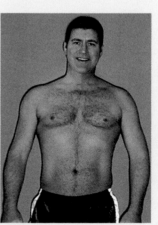

WEIGHT, WEEK 1: 212
WEIGHT, WEEK 6: 185

"From age 16 to 28 I weighed 145. I was a toothpick. A friend told me to enjoy it now, once you hit 30 that will all change. It did! Behind my back my own mother told my sister, 'I can't believe how big he got.' To quote her: 'Even his face looks fat.' Thanks to the Abs Diet, I no longer have a 'fat face' or body. I feel great and look better than I did at 16."

KNEE RAISE WITH DROP

Targets both the lower abs and obliques

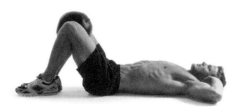

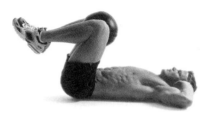

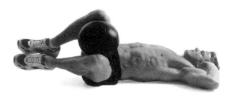

Lie on your back, with your hands behind your ears, knees bent, and feet on the floor. Position a medicine ball between your knees. Keep your lower back on the floor throughout the exercise. Contract your abdominals and pull your knees to your chest. Lower your knees to the left, bring them back to center, then return to the starting position. Drop your knees to the right on the next repetition, and alternate sides for each repetition.

12 repetitions [*Advanced*]

DOUBLE CRUNCH

Targets both the upper and lower abs

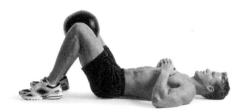

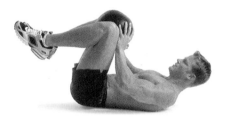

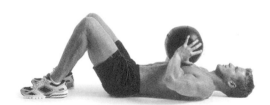

Lie on your back, with your knees bent and your feet on the floor. Position a medicine ball between your knees and rest your hands lightly on your chest. Exhale as you lift your shoulders off the floor and bring your knees to your chest. Grab the ball with your hands and bring it to your chest as you inhale and return your shoulders and legs to the starting position. Transfer the ball back to your legs on the next repetition, and keep alternating ball positions for the entire set.

12 repetitions [Advanced]

V-UP

Targets both the upper and lower abs

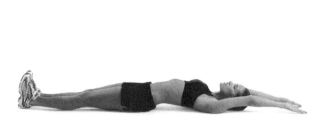
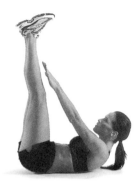

Lie on your back, with your legs and arms extended. Keeping your knees and elbows straight, simultaneously lift your upper body while trying to touch your fingers to your toes.

5–10 repetitions [*Advanced*]

DOUBLE CRUNCH WITH A CROSS

Targets both the upper and lower abs plus the obliques

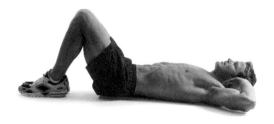
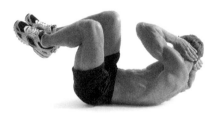

Lie on your back with your knees bent, your feet flat on the floor, your head and neck relaxed, and your hands behind your ears. Use your lower abs to lift both knees, and cross them toward your left shoulder as you simultaneously use your upper abs to raise your left shoulder and cross it toward your right knee. Hold for a second. Lower your legs and torso to the starting position and repeat to the other side.

10 repetitions each side [*Advanced*]

TRAVIS THOMSEN

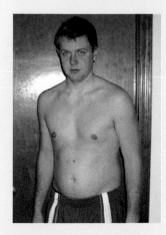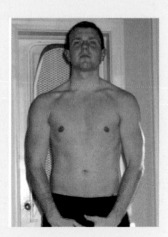

WEIGHT, WEEK 1: 194
WEIGHT, WEEK 6: 176

"Manhattan on the rocks. Years later I would come to hate those words, as diabetes soldiered through my uncle's body, remnants of bourbon aiding the process. Collegiate years of binge drinking drove me 30 pounds overweight. I needed a change. The Abs Diet provided that opportunity—a reason, as if I needed one, to better myself. I have not only altered my appearance but given myself a chance to live a little longer."

MEET YOUR MUSCLES

Don't you think you ought to know what you've been working?

CHEST: PUT UP A GREAT FRONT

The pectoralis major, the larger layer and the one lying closer to the skin, is divided into three parts: the clavicular, which starts high at the collarbone; the abdominal, which originates at your external oblique muscles; and the sternocostal, which starts at the breastbone. Each stretches across your chest in a fan shape, starting wide at the center of your body, then tapering at the side of your body to attach to the top of the humerus—the bone in your upper arm. The pectoralis minor is a thinner, more triangular muscle that lies beneath the pectoralis major. It starts along the third, fourth, and fifth ribs and stretches to connect to the shoulder blade. It is largely used to pull up on the ribs during heavy breathing. Together, the pectoralis major and pectoralis minor are responsible for rotating your upper arms and moving them across your body horizontally, as well as flexing the shoulder joints.

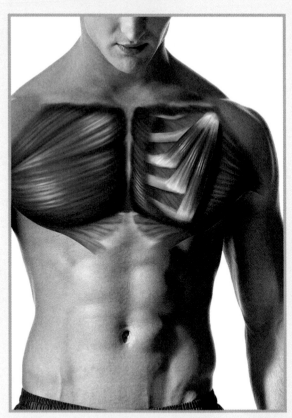

What Are They Good For?

- **More power:**
A strong chest makes it easier to push off opponents in such contact sports as football, basketball, martial arts, and hockey.

- **Stronger swing:**
Forehand strokes in tennis and sidearm throws in baseball depend on chest strength for velocity.

- **Knockout punch:**
The chest moves your arms forward, so developing chest strength delivers more power toward a target.

- **Better sex:**
A stronger, bigger chest gives men more strength and support in bed.

- **More lift:**
For women, stronger chest muscles can accentuate appearances.

BICEPS: THE BULGES EVERYONE WILL NOTICE

The biceps brachii muscle covers the front part of your upper arm and has two sections, or heads (the prefix "bi" means "two"). The long head—also called the outer head—attaches by way of the biceps tendon to the scapula, or shoulder blade, at the glenoid cavity deep inside the shoulder capsule. The short head stems from a bony hook (the coracoid) near the top of the scapula. The two muscles join below the shoulder, and their combined end attaches to the radius, one of the two major bones of the forearm.

The brachialis is sandwiched between the humerus (the upper arm bone) and the biceps. Developing this deep muscle gives it no place to go but up, pushing the biceps higher. Together the biceps and the brachialis are responsible for flexing your forearm toward your upper arm and turning your palm and forearm up.

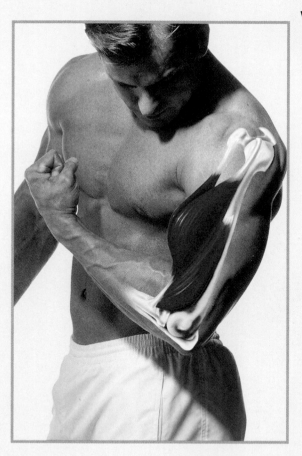

What Are They Good For?

• **Stronger grip:**
Nearly all biceps exercises strengthen tendons and muscles in your wrists.

• **Perfect stride:**
Since you pump your arms as you run, strong biceps add support to help you improve your pace.

• **Attention getter:**
It's one of the few muscles you can expose almost anywhere. Sculpted arms make others inclined to assume the rest of you is chiseled as well.

• **V shape:**
Back exercises require help from your biceps. The stronger the biceps, the more weight you can handle during back exercises.

• **Great sex:**
For men, certain sexual positions (like standing variations) mean you'll need well-built biceps to support her body.

UPPER BACK: GIMME A V!

The latissimus dorsi, the largest muscle of the back, is a broad, fan-shaped muscle that starts at the upper end of the humerus and runs down to attach low on the vertebral column and pelvic girdle. You have a lat on each side of your body; the muscle serves primarily to pull down the arm. It can also pull the body up toward the arm. For each of these tasks, the lats get assistance from the teres major—a muscle that runs from the outer edge of the scapula (shoulder blade) to the humerus. The trapezius muscles are long, triangle-shaped muscles that start at the base of the skull and attach to the backs of the collarbones and scapulae. They have several jobs, including scapular elevation (shrugging your arms up), scapular depression (pulling the shoulder blades down), and scapular adduction (pulling the shoulder blades together). Beneath the trapezius lie the rhomboid muscles, which also assist with scapular adduction.

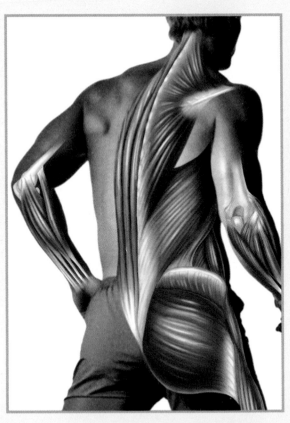

What Are They Good For?

• Harder throw:
Your back helps you rotate your upper arms, so strengthening your back gives your throws extra snap.

• Better posture:
A developed back helps prevent imbalances caused by an overdeveloped chest.

• More pulling power:
A stronger back adds strength to your swimming stroke and will help pull your body up when climbing—whether up a mountain or a ladder.

• Thinner waist:
Reshaping your uppper back to appear wider at the top helps create a V shape that makes your waistline appear smaller.

SHOULDERS: ROUND 'EM OUT

The anterior and middle deltoids originate on the collarbone, while the posterior deltoids start on the scapula (shoulder blade). All three sections come together and attach to the humerus. The main function of your deltoids is to move your arms away from your body, but each set of deltoid fibers has its own role. The anterior section raises your arms in front of your body; the middle section lifts them out to the sides; and the posterior section raises them behind you. Because they are located in both the front and the back of your body, deltoids act as the secondary movers during numerous exercises. The anterior deltoids assist the pectoral muscles in many chest exercises, while the posterior deltoids assist in many upper-back exercises that involve the teres major, rhomboids, and trapezius.

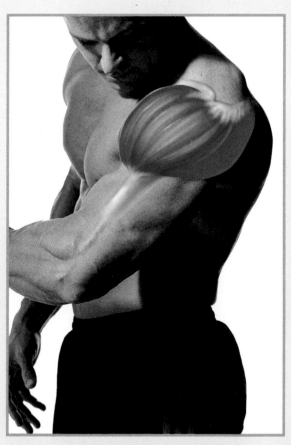

What Are They Good For?

• **More power:**
Because of their connection to other muscles, stronger shoulders give you extra strength in every exercise that works your chest, back, and arms.

• **Injury prevention:**
The posterior deltoids are responsible for decelerating your arms every time you throw or swing. Not being able to effectively slow down your arms places more stress on elbow joints.

• **Good posture:**
Keeping the three parts of the shoulders strong helps stabilize your shoulder girdle and keep your shoulders in alignment.

• **Stronger pull:**
Your shoulders share the responsibility of pulling your arms behind your body, giving you extra power for swimming or rowing.

TRICEPS: TIME TO GET STRONG-ARMED

The lateral head of this upper arm muscle attaches to the back of your humerus and forms the outer side of your triceps. It makes up most of the horseshoe shape of the muscle. The medial head is located along the middle of the back of your upper arm and also attaches to the humerus. The long head is located along the inside your arm and attaches to the scapula. All three heads connect to a tendon attached to the ulna (one of the two bones of the forearm). Together, the three heads are responsible for extending the elbow (straightening your arm). The long head also helps stabilize the underside of your shoulder joint, and it assists your upper-back muscles in arm adduction (bringing your arm down and in toward your body).

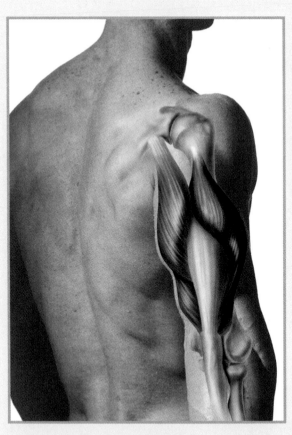

What Are They Good For?

• **Toned arms:**
Most of us target biceps, but the triceps make up 60 percent of the arms. Working your triceps gives you a more muscular and toned look.

• **More power:**
Throwing, punching, swinging, or pushing starts with your chest and ends with your triceps. Strong triceps provide an extra burst of strength when you straighten your arms.

• **Injury prevention:**
Triceps protect elbow joints by acting as shock absorbers, decreasing stress when your elbows are forced to flex suddenly.

• **Better body:**
Most chest and shoulder exercises rely heavily on the triceps as a secondary muscle to move weight. If you strengthen them, they won't give up before they should, so you'll achieve bigger gains with your chest and shoulder routines.

HAMSTRINGS: THE BICEPS OF YOUR LEGS

Your hamstrings are located on the back of your thighs and are made up of three separate muscle groups—the semimembranosus, semitendinosus, and biceps femoris. The first two muscles start on the ischial tuberosity (just beneath the gluteus maximus, on the pelvic bones) and attach to the medial tibia (the shin bone). The third muscle—the biceps femoris—has two heads. The long head starts on the ischial tuberosity, while the short head attaches to the femur (thigh bone). Both heads run down the back of the thigh and insert on the head of the fibula (the smaller bone on the lower leg). Separately, the three muscles help turn your knee inward and your feet outward. But together, they have two major functions: knee flexion (bending your knees) and hip extension (which happens whenever you kick a leg back). Other muscles assist your hamstrings in performing these two jobs. For instance, whenever you flex your knees, you also use your sartorious gracillus and gastrocnemius muscles. Whenever you extend your hips, your glutes and erector spinae muscles assist in the motion.

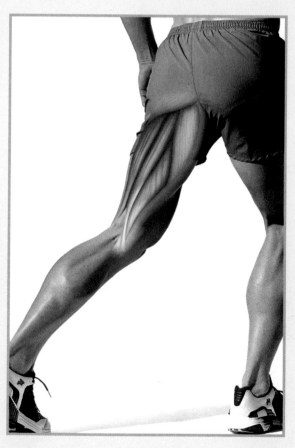

What Are They Good For?

• **Stronger strides:**
Your hamstrings pull your heels back toward your butt, while your glutes extend your legs back. Training both can lengthen your stride and provide more power for each push-off.

• **Better balance:**
Many hamstring exercises also challenge your stability. The result is quicker recovery of lost balance.

• **Healthier knees:**
Your anterior cruciate ligaments (ACLs) rely on your hamstrings to help them stabilize the knees whenever the knees bend while decelerating. Having a strong set of hamstrings can help ACLs do their job and lower your risk of injury.

• **Amazing sex:**
Having well-conditioned hamstrings and glutes makes it easier for a man to curl his pelvis forward to meet a woman halfway when she's on top. That can increase pleasure for him and her.

QUADRICEPS: A LARGE ORDER OF THIGHS

The quadriceps, on the front of the thigh, are made up of four individual, interdependent muscles. The vastus intermedius attaches to and covers much of the front and sides of the femur (thigh bone), but it is not visible because it lies underneath the rectus femoris. The rectus femoris starts at the pelvis and runs down the thigh, in front of the vastus intermedius. The vastus lateralis and vastus medialis begin at the outer and inner sides of the top of the femur. All four muscles run down your thigh and converge at the patellar tendon, which attaches along the upper part of the tibia. Together, the four muscles are responsible primarily for extending your knees (straightening your legs), but they also help stabilize the inner and outer sides of your knee joints. Because many of the exercises that target the quadriceps also involve the lower legs, the quads often work in unison with the gastrocnemius and soleus muscles in your calves.

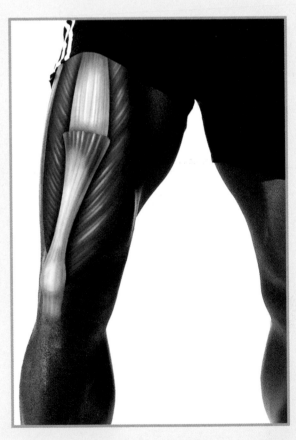

What Are They Good For?

• **More stamina:**
Many sports and activities require constant side-to-side movements, which work the quadriceps from the outside of the muscle to the inside. Strengthening your quads keeps them from tiring out.

• **Explosive takeoffs:**
Training the quads makes it easier to straighten the legs with more force, giving you more power whenever you use your legs to push forward or up.

• **More stability:**
Conditioning your quadriceps also strengthens the ligaments and tendons in your legs—critical elements that help support the knees. This in turns makes your knees more stable and less susceptible to injury.

• **Better sex:**
For men, thrusting forward while propped up on your knees requires a lot of hip flexion and hip extension. Strong quadriceps and hip flexors will help.

ABDOMINALS: TIME FOR A GUT CHECK

Your abdominals are composed of four muscle groups: the rectus abdominis, the external and internal obliques, and the transverse abdominis. Together, the four muscle groups support the torso and assist it in various movements—bending the body to either side, twisting right and left, and lowering and raising the upper body. The rectus abdominis, which is responsible for pulling your torso toward your hips, attaches to the sternum and your fifth through seventh ribs, and connects to your pubic bone. The external obliques run diagonally down from the lower ribs and connect to the pelvis and the pubic bone. The internal obliques, which lie underneath the external obliques and run diagonally to them, start on the iliac crest and connect to your lower three ribs. The internal and external obliques are responsible for torso rotation and lateral flexion (bending to the side). Lastly, the transverse abdominis muscle, which runs underneath your obliques, stretches from your lower ribs to your pubic bone. Its main job is to pull your abdominal wall inward, protecting your internal organs and helping you expel air.

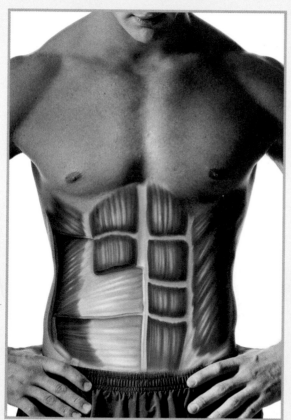

What Are They Good For?

- **Extra power:**
Exercising your abs muscles using moves that involve twisting can build the kind of rotational strength your midsection needs for delivering extra power when you throw, punch, or swing.

- **Better posture:**
Tight lower-back muscles from excessive running pull your spine out of natural alignments. Strengthening your abdominal wall can correct this muscular imbalance, improving your body's posture to allow it to function more efficiently.

- **Less pain:**
The weaker your abdominal muscles, the more your lower back has to compensate to support your body. Keeping the abs strong can balance the workload and protect your back from strains and pulls.

- **Better protection:**
Most abdominal exercises work the transverse abdominis, the thin band of muscle that supports and protects your internal organs.

LOWER BACK: YOUR BODY'S TRUE SUPPORT GROUP

The erector spinae—or spinal erectors—is a deep-muscle group running along both sides of the spinal column, from the iliac crest (the back of the pelvis) to the ribs, vertebrae, and skull. Each erector is made up of three separate vertical columns of muscle—the iliocostalis (farthest from the spine), longissimus (in the middle), and spinalis (closest to the spine). Each of these three muscles is divided into three segments, each named for one of four locations along the spinal column: the captis (nearest the skull); cervicis (in the neck), thoracis (in the midback), or lumborum (in the lower back). Together, they work to extend the spine (straightening it after it's been flexed forward) and bend it posteriorly (arching your back). They also help to support your spinal column and assist with the extension and rotation of your head.

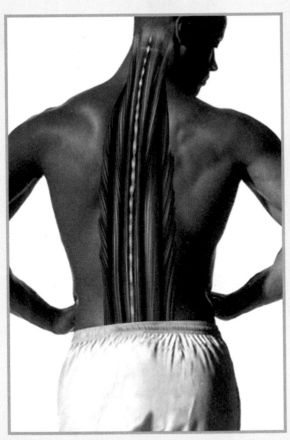

What Are They Good For?

• **More strength:**
Pulling, swinging, and throwing hard all rely on transferred power that comes from twisting your torso. Building up your lower-back muscles reinforces your core so your waist can deliver more twisting power.

• **Bigger muscles:**
The stronger your lower-back muscles are, the more supportive they'll be during exercises that work other muscles.

• **More energy:**
A stronger spine allows you to eliminate unnecessary steps or motions as you move. A healthy lower back can help your body perform tasks with less effort and fatigue.

• **Flatter stomach:**
Standing straight requires strong, resilient muscles along the spine and throughout the lower back. The stronger the muscles are, the more they'll minimize slouching, which pushes your stomach out.

Chapter 3

ABS3: STRENGTH TRAINING

To See the Biggest Results, You Have to Work Your Biggest Muscles

TO SHOW OFF YOUR ABS, YOU HAVE TO BURN FAT. To burn fat, you have to build muscle (and resist the mashed potatoes). Remember that adding just one pound of muscle will force your body to burn up to an additional 50 calories a day, every day. So to maximize your muscle growth, this workout emphasizes the larger muscle groups of your body—chest, back, and legs. Yes, your legs. Most of us (men especially) ignore our legs in workouts the way sunglassed celebs ignore photographers. But your lower body is where you'll build the most muscle in the least amount of time; working this giant muscle mass triggers the release of large amounts of growth hormone, which in turn stimulates muscle growth throughout your body, kicks your fat burners into overdrive, and gives you that washboard stomach you want—all in less time than it takes Paris Hilton to find a new boyfriend.

Doesn't sound possible? In one Norwegian study, men who focused on lower-body work gained more upper-body strength than did those who emphasized upper-body exercises in their workouts. That doesn't mean you'll ignore your upper body. With the upper-body workout, you'll also work your largest muscles—your chest, back, and shoulders—to burn more fat. If you follow this program, you'll notice more growth and definition throughout your whole body, and you'll begin to reshape your body.

To get that done, you'll do circuit training. That is, you'll perform one set of an exercise and then move immediately to the next exercise, with no more than 30 seconds of rest (or 1 minute in some cases). Follow the order of exercises I've listed on the following pages; that will allow you to work different areas from set to set. By alternating between body parts, you'll keep your body in constant work mode and be able to perform the movements back-to-back without rest. Here's why circuit training works so well: You save time, because you cut the amount of rest you need when you alternate muscle groups. More important, you keep your heart rate elevated throughout the workout, so you burn even more fat. And you also do compound exercises that work many muscles at once. Most of the following exercises actually work dozens—if not hundreds—of different muscles throughout your body. In fact, in the section that starts on page 164, I've listed special multi-muscle moves that work just about your entire body in one move.

Before we move to the workouts, all you have to do to follow this strength program long-term is follow these principles.

Beginners do two circuits, then move to three. If you're just starting, do circuits twice. Move from exercise to exercise with no more than 30 seconds of rest in between. When you complete one circuit, rest for 2 minutes, then complete the second circuit. After the first 2 weeks, when you've become comfortable doing two complete circuits during a workout, increase your workload to three circuits per workout.

Challenge yourself. In every exercise, use a weight that you can handle comfortably for the number of repetitions noted. When that gets too easy, increase the weight on each set by 10 percent or less. To challenge yourself, you can vary the grip on certain exercises or do them a little slower. And virtually every barbell exercise can be done with dumbbells. The key point to remember: Don't let yourself get too comfortable, or you'll stop seeing benefits.

Follow these programs or build your own. In the following pages, I've outlined more than a hundred different exercises. You can do the programs exactly as described. Or you can go to the end of the chapter where I've given you a menu of different exercises for different body parts so you can construct your own customized workout. If you like exercises from one program, swap them into another. Essentially, as long as you follow the principles of circuit training, compound exercises, and hitting the major muscle parts, you can build thousands of different adaptations to fit your own preferences.

Shake things up every 4 to 6 weeks. To keep yourself—and your muscles—from adapting too comfortably to any one program, change your routine every 4 to 6 weeks. Yes, you'll be increasing weight during each program as you get stronger, but to really stimulate muscle growth, you'll want to vary your patterns with new exercises and approaches.

> **ABS FACT**
>
> **135**
>
> Pounds the average guy can bench press

The Abs Diet Original Circuit

This circuit hits all of your major body parts—with a special emphasis on legs in the third workout of the week.

MONDAY:

Complete one set of each abs exercise*, then complete the rest of the circuit twice.

EXERCISE	REPETITIONS	REST	SETS
Traditional Crunch*	12–15	none	1
Bent-Leg Knee Raise*	12–15	none	1
Oblique V-Up*	10 each side	none	1
Bridge*	1 or 2	none	1
Back Extension*	12–15	none	1
Squat	10–12	30 seconds	2
Bench Press	10	30 seconds	2
Pulldown	10	30 seconds	2
Military Press	10	30 seconds	2
Upright Row	10	30 seconds	2
Triceps Pushdown	10–12	30 seconds	2
Leg Extension	10–12	30 seconds	2
Biceps Curl	10	30 seconds	2
Leg Curl	10–12	30 seconds	2

TUESDAY (OPTIONAL):
Light Cardiovascular Exercise Such as Walking (Try for 30 Minutes at a Brisk Pace)

WEDNESDAY:
Total-Body Strength Training Workout with Abs Emphasis
Complete one set of each abs exercise* once, then complete rest of circuit twice.

EXERCISE	REPETITIONS	REST	SETS
Standing Crunch*	12–15	none	1
Pulse-Up*	12	none	1
Saxon Side Bend*	6–10 each side	none	1
Side Bridge*	1 or 2 each side	none	1
Back Extension*	12–15	none	1
Squat	10–12	30 seconds	2
Bench Press	10	30 seconds	2
Pulldown	10	30 seconds	2
Military Press	10	30 seconds	2
Upright Row	10	30 seconds	2
Triceps Pushdown	10–12	30 seconds	2
Leg Extension	10–12	30 seconds	2
Biceps Curl	10	30 seconds	2
Leg Curl	10–12	30 seconds	2

THURSDAY (OPTIONAL):
Light Cardiovascular Exercise Such as Walking (Try for 30–45 Minutes at a Brisk Pace)

FRIDAY:
Total-Body Strength Training Workout, with Leg Emphasis
Repeat entire circuit twice.

EXERCISE	REPETITIONS	REST	SETS
Squat	10–12	30 seconds	2
Bench Press	10	30 seconds	2
Pulldown	10	30 seconds	2
Traveling Lunge	10–12 each leg	30 seconds	2
Military Press	10	30 seconds	2
Upright Row	10	30 seconds	2
Step-Up	10–12 each leg	30 seconds	2
Triceps Pushdown	10–12	30 seconds	2
Leg Extension	10–12	30 seconds	2
Biceps Curl	10	30 seconds	2
Leg Curl	10–12	30 seconds	2

SATURDAY (OPTIONAL):
Abs Workout Plus Interval Workout
Complete one set of each abs exercise, then choose one interval workout from the selection in Chapter 4.

EXERCISE	REPETITIONS	REST	SETS
Traditional Crunch	12–15	None	1
Bent-Leg Knee Raise	12	None	1
Oblique V-Up	6–10 each side	None	1
Bridge	1–2	None	1
Back Extension	12–15	None	1

SUNDAY: OFF

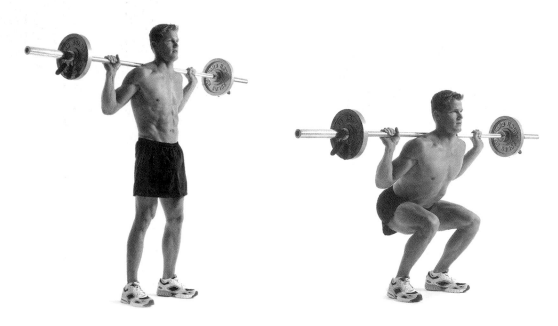

SQUAT

Hold a barbell behind you with an overhand grip, so that it rests comfortably on your upper back. Set your feet shoulder-width apart; keep your knees slightly bent, back straight, and eyes focused straight ahead. Slowly lower your body as if you were sitting back into a chair, keeping your back naturally aligned and your lower legs nearly perpendicular to the floor. When your thighs are parallel to the floor, pause, then return to the starting position.

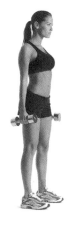
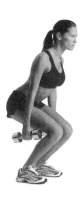

HOME VARIATION: *Same, but with one dumb-bell in each hand, your palms facing your outer thighs.*

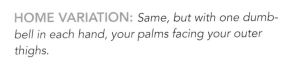

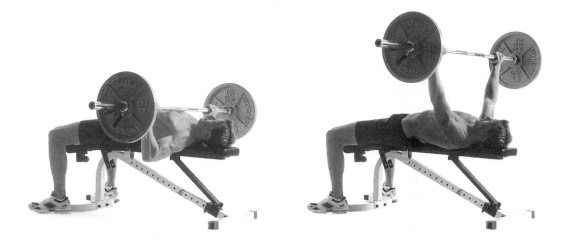

BENCH PRESS

Lie on your back on a flat bench with your feet on the floor. Grab the barbell with an overhand grip, your hands just a little more than shoulder-width apart. Lift the bar off the uprights and hold it at arm's length over your chest. Slowly lower the bar to your chest. Pause, then push the bar back to the starting position.

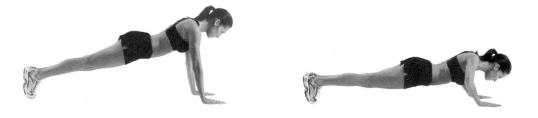

HOME VARIATION: *Do standard pushups: Get in a pushup position with your hands about shoulder-width apart. Bend at the elbows while keeping your back straight until your chin almost touches the floor, then push back up.*

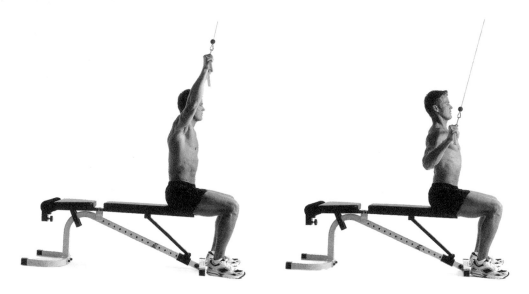

PULLDOWN

Stand facing a lat pulldown machine. Reach up and grasp the bar with an overhand grip that's 4 to 6 inches wider than your shoulders. Sit on the seat, letting the resistance of the bar extend your arms above your head. When you're in position, pull the bar down until it touches your upper chest. Hold this position for 1 second, then return to the starting position.

HOME VARIATION: *Bent-Over Row. Stand with your knees slightly bent and shoulder-width apart. Bend over so that your back is almost parallel to the floor. Holding a dumbbell in each hand, let your arms hang toward the floor. With your palms facing in, pull the dumbbells toward you until they touch the outside of your chest. Pause, then return to the starting position.*

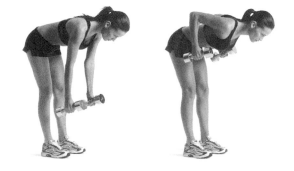

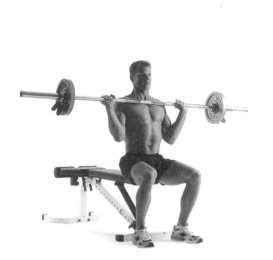
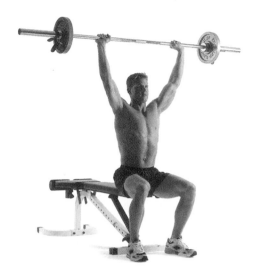

MILITARY PRESS

Sitting on an exercise bench, hold a barbell at shoulder height with your hands shoulder-width apart. Press the weight straight overhead so that your arms are almost fully extended, hold for a count of one, then bring it down to the front of your shoulders. Repeat.

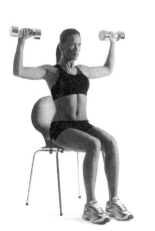
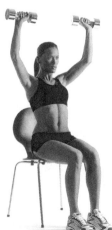

HOME VARIATION: *Sitting on a sturdy chair instead of a bench, hold one dumbbell in each hand, about level with your ears. Push the dumbbells straight overhead so that your arms are almost fully extended, hold for a count of one, then return to the starting position. Repeat.*

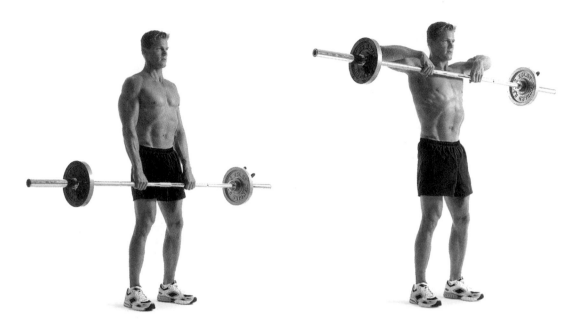

UPRIGHT ROW

Grab a barbell with an overhand grip and stand with your feet shoulder-width apart and your knees slightly bent. Let the barbell hang at arm's length on top of your thighs, thumbs pointed toward each other. Bending your elbows, lift your upper arms straight out to the sides; pull the barbell straight up until your upper arms are parallel to the floor and the bar is just below chin level. Pause, then return to the starting position.

HOME VARIATION: *Same, using one dumbbell in each hand.*

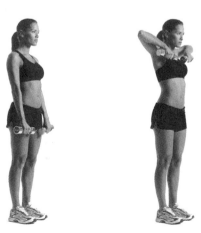

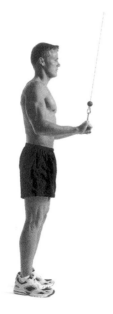
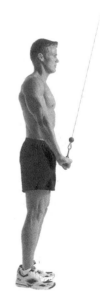

TRICEPS PUSHDOWN

While standing, grip a bar attached to a high pulley cable or lat machine with your hands about 6 inches apart. With your elbows tucked against your sides, bring the bar down until it is directly in front of you. With your forearms parallel to the floor (the starting position), push the bar down until your arms are extended straight down with the bar near your thighs. Don't lock your elbows. Return to the starting position.

HOME VARIATION: *Triceps Kickback. Stand with your knees slightly bent and shoulder-width apart. Bend over so that your back is almost parallel to the ground. Bend your elbows to about 90-degree angles, raising them to just above the level of your back. This is the starting position. Extend your forearms backward, keeping your upper arms stationary. When they're fully extended, your arms should be parallel to the ground. Pause, then return to the starting position.*

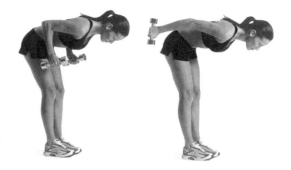

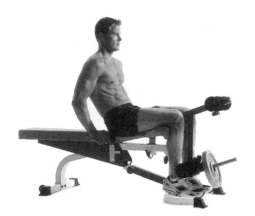 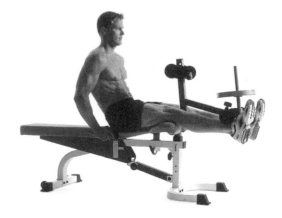

LEG EXTENSION

Sitting on a leg extension machine with your feet under the footpads, lean back slightly and lift the pads with your feet until your legs are extended.

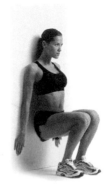

HOME VARIATION: *Squat Against the Wall.*
Stand with your back flat against a wall. Squat
down so that your thighs are parallel to the
ground. Hold that position for as long as you can.
That's one set. Aim for 20 seconds to start, and
work your way up to 45 seconds.

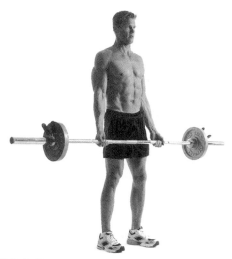
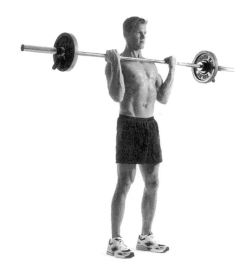

BICEPS CURL

Stand while holding a barbell in front of you, palms facing out, with your hands shoulder-width apart and your arms hanging in front of you. Curl the weight toward your shoulders, hold for 1 second, then return to the starting position.

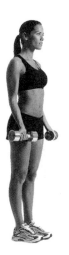
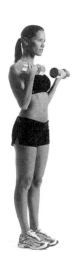

HOME VARIATION: *Same, using a set of dumb-bells instead.*

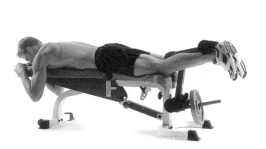

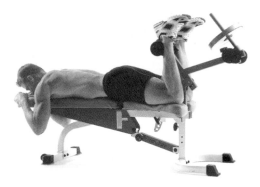

LEG CURL

Lie facedown on a leg curl machine and hook your ankles under the padded bar. Keeping your stomach and pelvis against the bench, slowly raise your feet toward your butt, curling up the weight until your feet nearly touch your butt. Slowly return to the starting position.

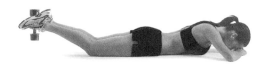

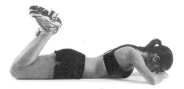

HOME VARIATION: *Lie down with your stomach on the floor. Put a light dumbbell between your feet (so that the top end of the dumbbell rests on the bottom of your feet). Squeeze your feet together and curl them up toward your butt.*

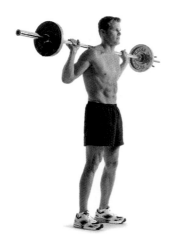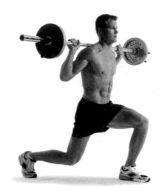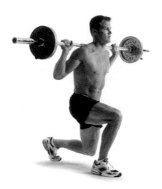

TRAVELING LUNGE

Hold a barbell across your upper back. Stand, with your feet hip-width apart, at one end of the room; you need room to walk about 20 steps. Step forward with your left foot, and lower your body so that your left thigh is parallel to the floor and your right thigh is perpendicular to the floor (your right knee should bend and almost touch the floor). Stand and bring your right foot up next to your left, then repeat with the right leg lunging forward.

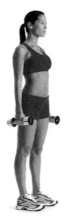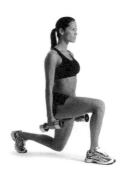

HOME VARIATION: *Use dumbbells, holding one in each hand with your arms at your sides. If you don't have enough space, do the move in one place, alternating your lead foot with each lunge.*

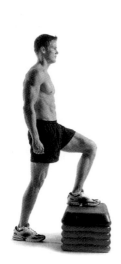
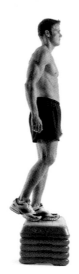
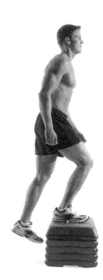

STEP-UP

Use a step or bench that's 18 inches off the ground. Place your left foot on the step so that your knee is bent at 90 degrees. Your knee should not advance past the toes of your left foot. Push off with your left foot, and bring your right foot onto the step, keeping your back straight. Now step down with the left foot, followed by the right. Alternate the leading foot, or do all of the repetitions leading with one foot and then alternating. Once you're comfortable, add dumbbells.

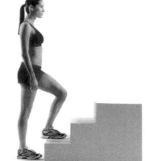
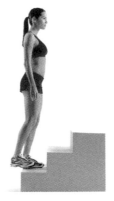
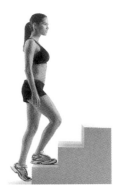

HOME VARIATION:
Same; if you don't have a step, use stairs.

The Sequel Workout: An Amazing Alternative

This workout is very like the original Abs Diet circuit but uses substitute exercises for each of the different muscle groups. You can switch to this circuit, or substitute favorite exercises to construct a hybrid circuit between this workout and the original circuit.

EXERCISE	REPETITIONS	REST	SETS
Incline Bench Press	10	30 seconds	2
Cable Row	10–12	30 seconds	2
Uneven Step Squats	6 each side	30 seconds	2
Lateral Raises	12–15	30 seconds	2
Dumbbell Upright Row and Shrug	12	30 seconds	2
Weight Plate Deadlift	10–12	30 seconds	2
Dumbbell Incline Curl	10 each arm	30 seconds	2
Triceps Extension	10–12	30 seconds	2

"THANKS, ABS DIET!"

TIM DUBOSE

WEIGHT, WEEK 1: 204
WEIGHT, WEEK 6: 190

"I ate, I stayed full, I built muscle, and I lost fat! What I eat and how I eat has changed forever, thanks to the Abs Diet."

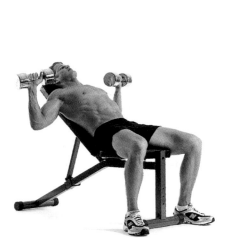
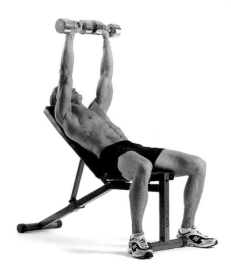

INCLINE BENCH PRESS

Grab a pair of dumbbells (or a barbell) and lie on an incline bench with your hips and thighs in a straight line and parallel to the floor. Press the weights straight up, then lower to your chest, and repeat.

"THANKS, ABS DIET!"

JEFF GARDE

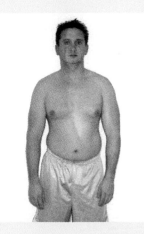
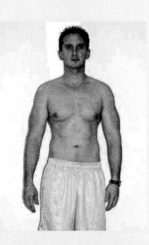

WEIGHT, WEEK 1: 160
WEIGHT, WEEK 6: 145

"I'm in better shape at 32 then when I was 18. I never thought I would say that. The program educated me on knowing what to eat, how often to eat, and the importance of exercising and weight training. I feel and look healthier then ever, which has given me more confidence, self-discipline, and a feeling of having control over my life again."

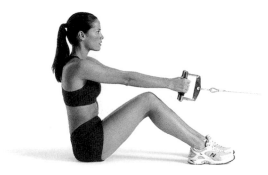
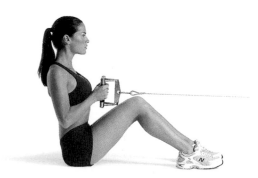

CABLE ROW

Sit on the floor and grasp the handles at the end of the cable, keeping your upper body straight and your knees slightly flexed. Pull the handles to your chest with your arms. Then return toward the starting position until your arms are straight.

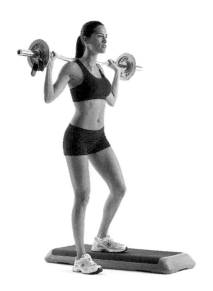
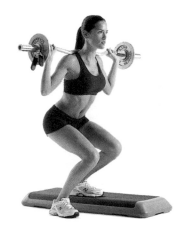

UNEVEN STEP SQUAT

Stand with a barbell resting on your upper back, with your left foot on an exercise step and your right foot to the right of the step. Lower your body until your right thigh is parallel to the floor. Pause, then return to the starting position. Do one set this way, then switch sides. (You can also hold dumbbells.)

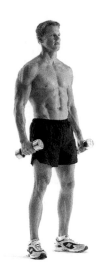
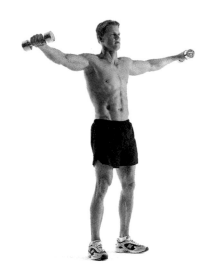

LATERAL RAISES

Stand with your feet shoulder-width apart and your arms at your sides. Hold a dumbbell in each hand with your palms facing your body and your elbows slightly bent. Raise both dumbbells straight out from your sides until they're at shoulder level. Pause, then lower.

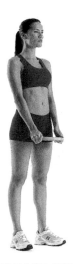
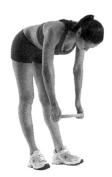

WEIGHT PLATE DEADLIFT

Stand with a light weight plate in both hands. Bend your knees slightly. Keeping your back straight, slowly bend forward from the hips as far as you can, lowering the plate to the floor. Your arms remain straight during the exercise. Slowly rise into the starting position.

VARIATION 1: *Stand on a step and let the plate extend beyond the level of your feet. Put your heels together and point your toes out like a duck. This will give your glutes more of a workout.*

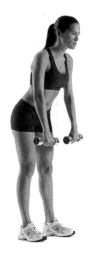
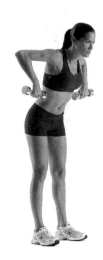

DUMBBELL UPRIGHT ROW AND SHRUG

Hold a pair of dumbbells with an overhand grip and let them hang at arm's length in front of your thighs. Bend forward from your waist at about 10 degrees. Keep your forearms pointed down as you lift your upper arms until they're parallel to the floor. At the same time, shrug your shoulders up as if you were trying to touch them to your ears. Pause, then slowly return to the starting position.

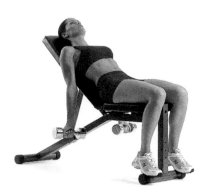
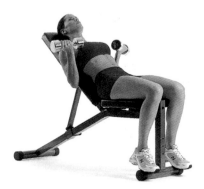

DUMBBELL INCLINE CURL

Set an incline bench at a 45-degree angle. Grab a pair of dumbbells and lie faceup on the bench. Let your arms hang straight down from your shoulders and turn your palms forward. Keeping your upper arms still, slowly curl the weight up as high as you can using only your forearms. Then, without pausing, take 5 seconds to gradually lower the dumbbells to the starting position.

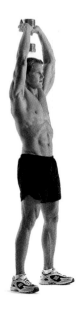 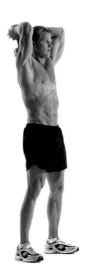

TRICEPS EXTENSION

Hold a single dumbbell at one end with both hands and press it overhead. Keep your elbows close to your ears as you lower the dumbbell slowly behind your head. Keep your upper arms vertical—only your forearms should move. Extend the dumbbell smoothly back to the top position.

"THANKS, ABS DIET!"

MICHAEL MASTERFIELD

WEIGHT, WEEK 1: 191
WEIGHT, WEEK 6: 181

"After several attempts and failures at trying to get into shape, I was convinced that I would have to submit myself to a supplement-packed diet. But after I discovered and read *The Abs Diet*, I began to eat and exercise as the diet suggested. The fat just kept peeling away as the muscle made its appearance. Now I look good, feel good, and can't wait for the next 6 weeks."

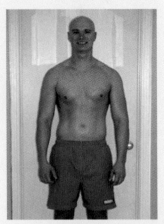

After

ABS DIET SUCCESS STORY

"BEING OUT OF SHAPE WAS A SMACK IN THE FACE"

Name: Richard Langdon

Age: 27

Height: 6'1"

Starting weight: 213

Six weeks later: 185

Starting waist size: 39

Six weeks later: 32

"It sounds kinda funny," Richard Langdon says, "but I was sitting on the couch and looked down and noticed I had a stomach and never really had that before." At that point, Langdon was already close to exceeding the maximum weight limit for the military, and he was watching guys nearly 10 years older than him beat him in physical tests.

"One of the hardest things was being only 26 and having people older than I am run faster than I was running and do a lot more than I was able to do," he says. "Looking at somebody 33 or 35 putting out more than me was like a smack in the face."

So Langdon decided to try the Abs Diet, ate the Powerfoods, used smoothies to satisfy sweet cravings, and worked out. He dropped weight—but the biggest thing he noticed was his energy level.

"I wasn't really tired anymore. Before, I'd get up at 6, and around 10:30 or 11, I'd get real tired, get something to eat, sit in my office and basically want to fall asleep at my desk," he says. "Since I lost the weight, I get up at 4, go all day long without any problems until I go to bed at 8 or 9 at night. I have more energy."

Since then, he's noticed a difference in not only his physical-test scores but also his self-esteem. ("I love to work out now; it's like a religion.") But his biggest surprise was that his total-body change even included his taste buds.

"I don't miss the sweets and the junk food," he says. "I really don't miss it. It sounds weird, but I crave vegetables now the same way I used to crave a Snickers or can of soda."

The No-Weights, No-Problem Workout: Blast Your Body

Sometimes, life doesn't allow you to have access to a gym or even a good set of weights—when you're on vacation, perhaps, or serving 20 in solitary. But you can use nature's best barbell—your own body. In fact, many athletes use their own body weight for hard-core workouts because it provides more than enough resistance when you're doing body-weight exercises. This circuit works all of your muscles, and you never have to lift a weight—except your own.

EXERCISE	REPETITIONS	REST	SETS
Broad Jump	10–12	30 seconds	2
Diamond Pushup	10–12	30 seconds	2
Reaching Lunge	6–8 each leg	30 seconds	2
Bench Dip	10–12	30 seconds	2
Skiing Wall Squat	5	30 seconds	2
Donkey Kick	15 each leg	30 seconds	2
Boot Slappers	8	30 seconds	2
Shadow Boxing	50 punches	1 minute	2

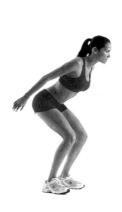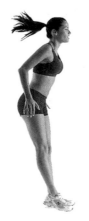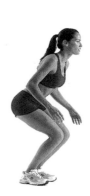

BROAD JUMP

Stand with your feet shoulder-width apart and knees slightly bent. Dip your knees and jump forward as far as you can. Land on both feet with flexed knees. Pause, turn around, then jump back. Complete a set of 10.

VARIATION 1: *As soon as your toes touch the floor after the jump, jump again immediately.*

VARIATION 2: *After each broad jump, squat slightly and quickly explode straight up, reaching both arms overhead. Land with flexed knees, then jump forward again.*

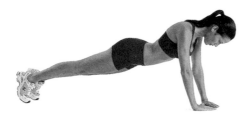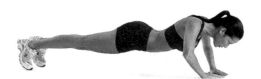

DIAMOND PUSHUP

Get into traditional pushup position, but place your hands directly under your chest with your index fingers and thumbs spread and touching; that's the diamond. Keep your back flat throughout the movement. Lower your body until your chest nearly touches your hands. Pause, then push your body back up to the starting position.

VARIATION 1: *If the move is too difficult, put your knees on the ground.*

VARIATION 2: *Elevate your feet on a bench, chair, or bed.*

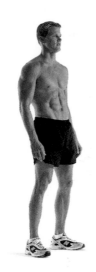 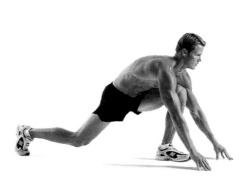

REACHING LUNGE

Stand with your feet shoulder-width apart. In one motion, take a lunging step forward as far as you can with your left foot and reach forward with both hands to touch the floor in front of you. Quickly reverse the motion to return to the starting position, then switch legs.

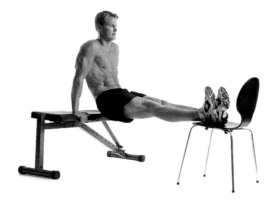 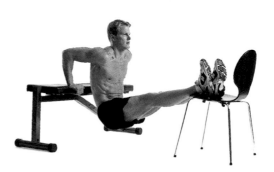

BENCH/CHAIR DIP

Place your hands behind you on the edge of a bench or chair and your feet on another bench or chair (or the floor) a few feet in front of you. Lower your body until your upper arms are nearly parallel to the floor. Pause, then press back to the starting position.

VARIATION: *Ask someone to add a weight plate, phone book, or your carry-on for extra resistance.*

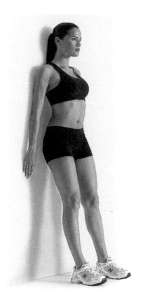
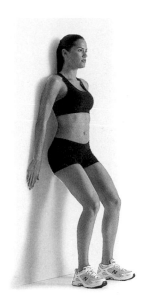
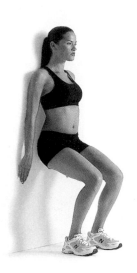
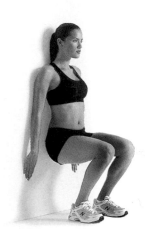

SKIING WALL SQUAT

Lean against a wall, with your feet 18 to 24 inches away from it and shoulder-width apart. Bend your knees slightly and hold that position for 5 to 10 seconds. Bend deeper and hold. Repeat until you've hit five different positions; go as low as you can.

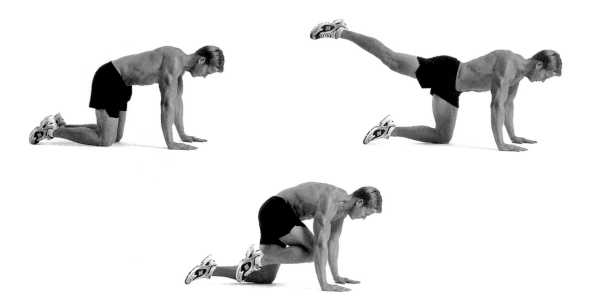

DONKEY KICK

Get down on your hands and knees and kick your right leg back and up as high as you can. Finish by arching your back and pulling your knee to your chest. Repeat on the other side.

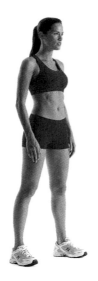 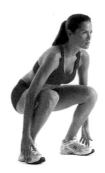

BOOT SLAPPERS

Stand with your legs slightly wider than shoulder-width, squat down, slap the sides of your ankles, then stand back up. Repeat 10 to 20 times.

VARIATION: *After you slap your ankles, explode and jump straight up instead of standing up.*

"THANKS, ABS DIET!"

CHAD WILLIAMS

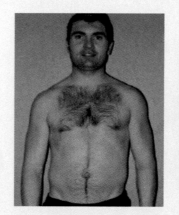 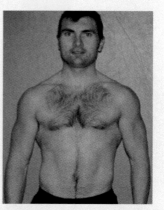

WEIGHT, WEEK 1: 184
WEIGHT, WEEK 6: 174

"This program was great for changing my body and my lifestyle. I went from regularly exercising in my early 20s to intermittent exercise by age 30. I was wearing BBPs (big boy pants, as my wife calls them), which was tough. I'm now proud to say I have made a permanent change in my body and outlook because this diet is so easy to live with. Thank you! I've sworn off the BBPs for good!"

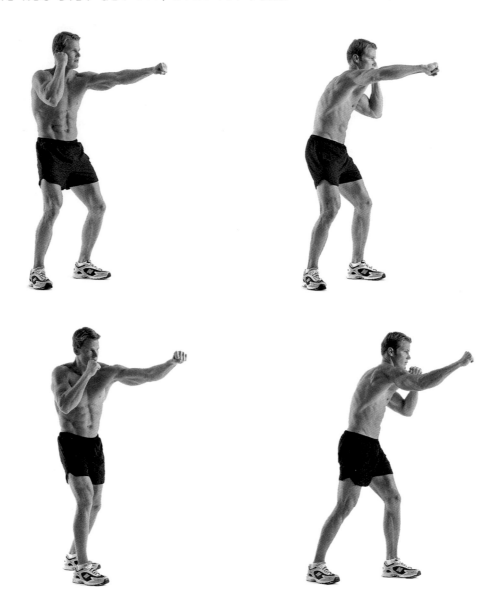

SHADOW BOXING

Throw punches while bobbing on your feet like a boxer: 10 left jabs, 10 right jabs, 10 left hooks, 10 right hooks, 10 left uppercuts, 10 right uppercuts. See page 223 for punch descriptions.

The Fight Club Workout: It Really Packs a Punch

Normally, I don't recommend fighting—unless your opponent is air. However, using martial-arts moves can be a fantastic way to get a resistance workout if you don't have access to weights or the time to get to the gym. Do this heart-raising workout, which will also work the muscles in your upper and lower body. First, do the Warm-Up Move on the next page for 5 minutes, then complete the following circuit 2 to 4 times.

1. Lunge and Front Kick: 12 each leg

2. Warm-Up Move: 1 minute

3. Turn, Block, and Punch: 12 each arm

4. Warm-Up Move: 1 minute

5. Head Crusher: 12 each leg

6. Warm-Up Move: 1 minute

7. Pushup variation of choice (see pages 87, 105, 135, 152, 154, 157, 161, 193, 196, 197, 200, and 230): 12 to 15

8. Warm-Up Move: 1 minute

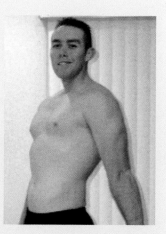

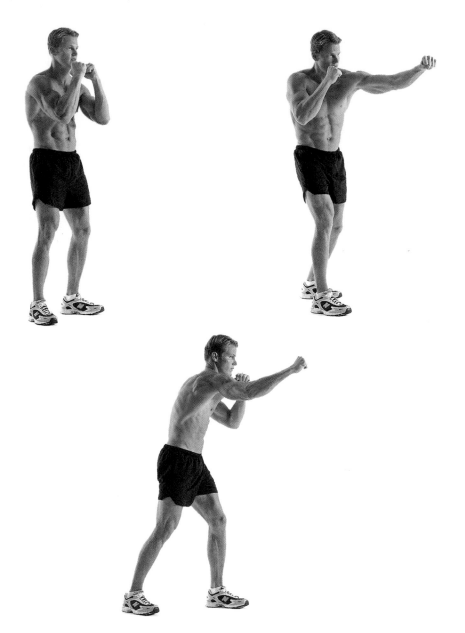

WARM-UP MOVE

Assume the starting position, which you'll use for all moves. Stand on the balls of your feet with your knees bent and your fists clenched at chin height. With your arms up, throw a punch with your left hand at chin height while you quickly step forward with your right foot and back with your left. Next punch with your right hand and switch the position of your feet.

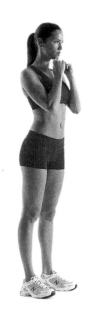

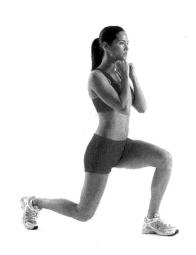

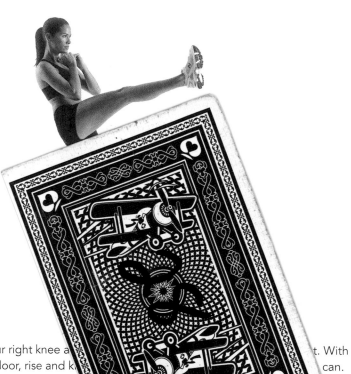

LUNGE AND FRONT KICK

Step back into a deep lunge, so your right knee a[...]t. With your left foot firmly planted on the floor, rise and k[...] can. Return to the standing position and repeat, steppin[...]

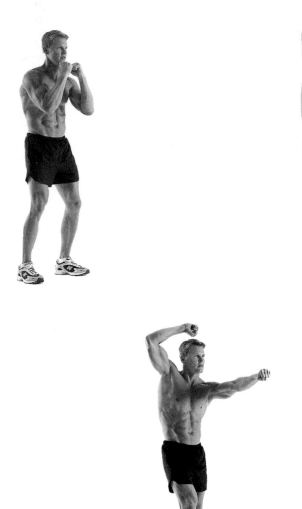

TURN, BLOCK, AND PUNCH

From the starting position, step back with either leg while lifting your right forearm above your head as if to block a punch. Now punch with your left hand. Resume the starting position and repeat the maneuver, stepping back with either leg and punching with your right hand.

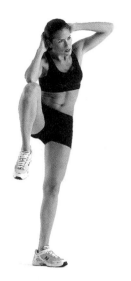
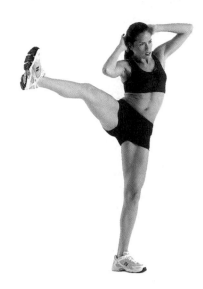

HEAD CRUSHER

Bring your right knee up and drop your right elbow down until they meet. Bend your torso slightly to the left to crunch your obliques. Kick your right foot out to the side, then snap it back. Return to the starting position and repeat the move, kicking with your left foot.

"THANKS, ABS DIET!"

BILL SCHNAKENBERG

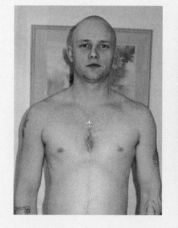
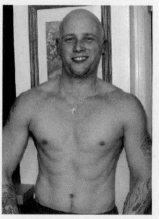

WEIGHT, WEEK 1: 170
WEIGHT, WEEK 6: 162

"In February my fiancée told me I was getting a beer belly, and it mortified me. I didn't think I could get rid of it in 6 weeks, but with a great diet plan and regular exercise, it paid off."

The Genius Dumbbell Workout: It's in Your Hands Now

Dumbbells may be even more useful than a Wet-Nap at a rib joint. They're small, so you can move them around from one area to another. They're easy to store, so you can exercise at home. They're versatile, so you can work every body part with them. And they're effective: Using dumbbells, you work parts of your body separately (which means the stronger side can't compensate for the weaker, as can happen with barbells). You can substitute dumbbells for most barbell moves throughout the book, or try this dumbbell-specific circuit.

EXERCISE	REPETITIONS	REST	SETS
Single-Leg Squat	8–12 each leg	30 seconds	2
Dumbbell Clean	10 each side	30 seconds	2
Clock Lunges	7 each side	30 seconds	2
Pushup Position Row	6 each arm	30 seconds	2
Overextension Kickback	8 each arm	30 seconds	2
Supinating Dumbbell Curl	8–12 each arm	30 seconds	2
Bentover Row with Back Extension	8	30 seconds	2
Dumbbell Lunge with Lateral Raise	6 each leg	30 seconds	2
Golf Squat	10–15 each side	30 seconds	2

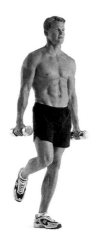
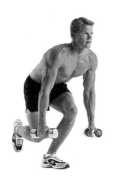

SINGLE-LEG SQUAT

Holding two dumbbells, stand with your knees slightly bent and your feet shoulder-width apart. Lift your right leg so that your knee is bent 90 degrees and your lower leg is parallel to the ground behind you. Slowly lower your body until your left thigh is parallel to the ground. Pause, then push your body back to the starting position. Finish all of the repetitions, then switch legs and repeat.

"THANKS, ABS DIET!"

GREG COYLE

WEIGHT, WEEK 1: 240
WEIGHT, WEEK 6: 217

"In December, my son turned 10, only 4 years younger than I was when my father died of diabetic and cardiac complications. I was getting heavy, out of shape, and tired all the time. Following the Abs Diet, I was able to regain the strength and muscle tone I have not had in 10 years. I learned how to eat well and work out effectively. The Abs Diet proved to be the fountain of youth."

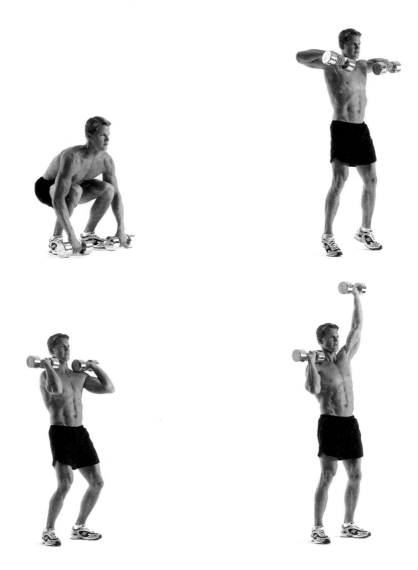

SINGLE-ARM DUMBBELL CLEAN

Squat over a pair of dumbbells and grab them with an overhand grip. Stand and lift both weights up to chest height. Quickly drop underneath the weights and "catch" them on your shoulders, with your elbows high. Drop your elbows, keeping the dumbbells at shoulder level. Push the dumbbell in your left hand straight up. Pause, then lower the dumbbell. Repeat the exercise, this time pressing up the weight in your right hand only.

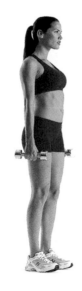
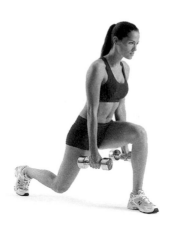
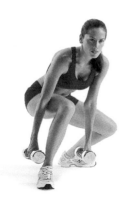
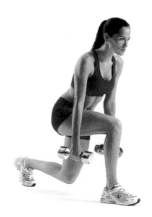

CLOCK LUNGE

Stand with your feet hip-width apart and hold dumbbells at your sides. Step backward with your right leg to 6 o'clock, until your right knee is just above the floor and your left thigh is parallel to the floor, keeping your left knee over (not past) your toes. Push back up to the starting position and repeat, this time stepping your right leg out to the side to 3 o'clock, keeping your toes pointed out to the side. Return to the starting position once more, then step once more, this time placing your foot forward to 12 o'clock. Return to the start position, then switch positions and step back with your left leg, moving to 6 o'clock, 3 o'clock, and 12 o'clock.

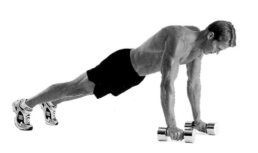
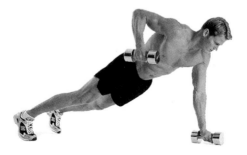

PUSHUP POSITION ROW

Get into pushup position with your arms straight and your hands resting on light dumbbells. Spread your feet apart for balance. Tighten your abs as you pull one dumbbell off the floor and draw it toward your chest until your elbow is above your back. Pause, then slowly return the weight to the floor and repeat with the other arm. TIP: If holding both dumbbells feels awkward, try doing the exercise holding only one dumbbell and place your other hand on the floor.

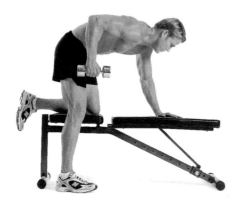
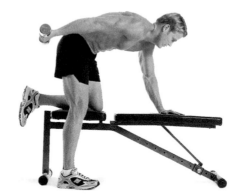

OVEREXTENSION KICKBACK

Grab a dumbbell in your right hand and place your left hand and knee on a bench. Place your right foot flat on the floor and bend forward at the hips so your torso is parallel to the floor. Bend your right arm at a 90-degree angle so that your upper arm is parallel with the floor (palm facing your leg). Without moving your upper arm, straighten your arm behind you. As the weight clears your butt, slowly rotate your palm up toward the ceiling so that the back of your hand faces your body when your arm is straightened. Pause, then slowly return to the starting position. TIP: If twisting the weight at the top of the movement feels awkward on your wrists, just do the move without the twist.

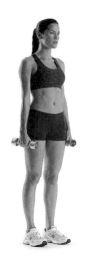 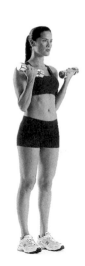

SUPINATING DUMBBELL CURL

Hold dumbbells at your sides, palms toward you. Curl the weights up, rotating your wrists inward 90 degrees by the time the weights reach your shoulders. Reverse this motion as you lower the weights.

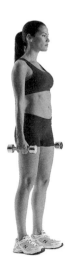 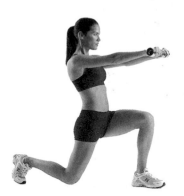

DUMBBELL LUNGE WITH FRONT RAISE

Stand holding a pair of dumbbells at your sides. Lunge forward with one foot as you raise your arms out to the front. Once your front knee is at a 90-degree angle (over your toes) and your arms are parallel to the floor, lower the weights, then push yourself back to the starting position. Repeat the move, this time lunging forward with the opposite leg.

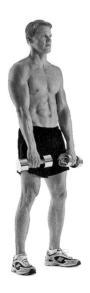

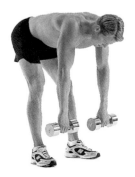

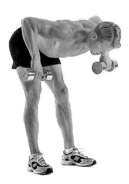

BENT-OVER ROW WITH BACK EXTENSION

Stand with your knees flexed and hold a pair of dumbbells at arm's length by your thighs, with your palms facing behind you. Bend forward at the hips until your torso is almost parallel to the floor and the weights are hanging directly beneath your shoulders. Now pull the dumbbells up toward your chest until your elbows extend pass your torso. Keep your arms stationary as you return to a standing position. Lower your arms and repeat.

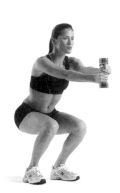
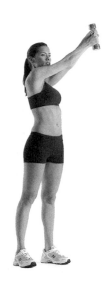

GOLF SQUAT

Hold one dumbbell with both hands at arm's length in front of your body. Keep your torso upright and lower your hips until your thighs are at least parallel to the floor. Pause 1 second, then rise to a standing position as you rotate your upper body to the left and lift the weight toward the ceiling, keeping your arms straight as if swinging a golf club. Lower the weight as you return the starting position. Repeat, this time rotating to your right.

"THANKS, ABS DIET!"

GLENN EUBINAG

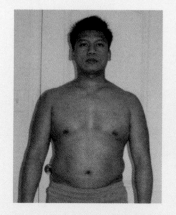
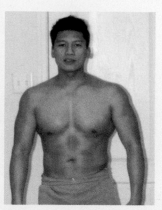

WEIGHT, WEEK 1: 168
WEIGHT, WEEK 6: 152

"At age 38 and after years of neglect, my 34-inch waist kept growing with no end in sight. I was astonished to see such dramatic results on the Abs Diet program. In only 6 weeks, I've been able to reduce to a 31-inch waist, and I feel like a million bucks. My wife has also taken a liking to my new, flat stomach."

The One-Weight Workout: Break Your Limits

If you work out at home, you probably don't have the space to rack 10 pairs of various weights of dumbbells to use for different exercises and body parts. You may own just one pair. This simple, 3-move circuit will allow you to work multiple body parts using the same pair of dumbbells—preferably medium-weight, approximately 20 to 25 pounds for men and 10 to 15 pounds for women. These three moves will work most of your major muscles, but, as an option, you can add one set of pushups and squats or lunges at the beginning or end of the circuit.

EXERCISE	REPETITIONS	REST	SETS
Single-Arm Row	12 each arm	30 seconds	4–5
Single-Arm Press and Bend	12 each arm	30 seconds	4–5
Side-Loaded Squat	12 each arm	30 seconds	4–5

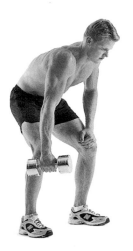 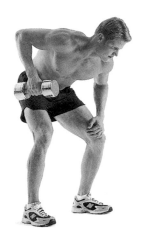

SINGLE-ARM ROW

Stand with your knees slightly bent and hold a dumbbell in your right hand with your palm facing your body. Lean forward at the hips until your torso is at a 45-degree angle. Pull the dumbbell to just below your rib cage, then lower it to the starting position. At the end of the set, switch arms.

VARIATION: *Perform the move on one leg. Stand on your right leg and lift your left leg in front as you lean over and row.*

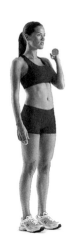
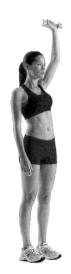
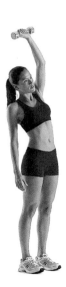

SINGLE-ARM PRESS AND BEND

Stand holding a dumbbell above your left shoulder in your left hand. Press the dumbbell up until your arm is straight. Tilt to your right side. Pause and return to the starting position. At the end of the set, switch arms.

VARIATION 1: *Dip your knees slightly. Quickly push the dumbbell up while standing up. Pause, then lower the weight.*

VARIATION 2: *Same as Variation 1, but jump in an explosive movement. Land on both feet, but with your opposite foot forward (left if the dumbbell is in your right hand) and leg slightly bent and back leg straight.*

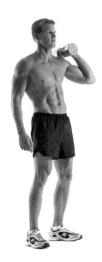

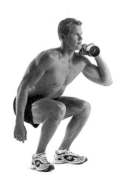

SIDE-LOADED SQUAT

Stand holding the dumbbell in your left hand at shoulder height. Lower your body until your thighs are parallel to the floor. Pause, then push back up to the starting position. At the end of the set, switch arms.

VARIATION 1: *Hold the dumbbell above your head with both hands in the center in an overhand grip, arms straight. Keep your shoulder blades pulled back as you squat.*

VARIATION 2: *Step forward with your left leg until your left thigh is parallel to the floor, while holding the dumbbell overhead with both hands. Then, with the same foot, step back into a reverse lunge. That counts as 2 repetitions.*

"THANKS, ABS DIET!"

COREY BUTTON

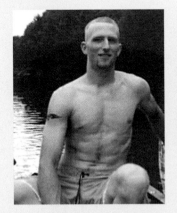

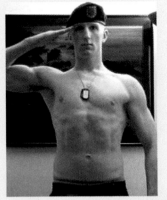

WEIGHT, WEEK 1: 189
WEIGHT, WEEK 6: 173

"Taking into account the right foods to eat to be able to define my body and especially my abs, along with exercise, has been huge in helping me reach my goals. This program showed me what to do, and the results are undeniable."

The Cage-Match Workout: Do It Faster, Get It Faster

Cages aren't just great for zoo animals and in-laws; they're also a great way to work out without having to wait for a dumbbell like you're in line at the deli counter. Cages allow you to do multiple exercises within a confined area; they're becoming popular in gyms as well as for home workouts. You can perform this entire workout with the cage system. You'll use the same approach as in your other circuits—you'll work major body parts and move from muscle to muscle quickly so that you can affect the most amount of muscle in the least time. The superset means that you do both exercises in the pair back-to-back without rest. Then rest for a minute and repeat the superset until you finish three sets of each exercise. Or move through the supersets like a circuit—do the first two exercises, rest, then the next two, and so on.

EXERCISE	REPETITIONS	REST	SETS
Superset 1:			
Dumbbell Lunge	10	0	3
Incline Press	10	1 minute	3
Superset 2:			
Pullup variation of choice (see pages 159 and 206)	max	0	3
Crunch variation of choice (see pages 23, 27, 30, 34–7, 39, 41, 43, 45, 52, 57–60, 63, 66, 69, 70, 150, or 193)	15	1 minute	3
Solo Set:			
Dumbbell Press	10	1 minute	3
Superset 3:			
Incline Dumbbell Curl	10	0	3
Dip	10	1 minute	3

WORK OUT AT HOME OR GYM?

My take: Work out wherever you're most likely to stick to your program. But you may see greater gains at the gym. Researchers found that men are able to bench-press an average of 41 pounds more with spectators than when they lift alone. The reason? The audience can be a huge motivator.

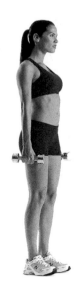
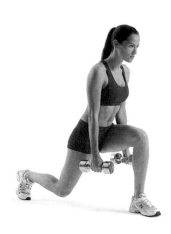

DUMBBELL LUNGE

Hold a dumbbell in each hand. Step forward with your right leg and lower your body until your front knee is bent 90 degrees and your left knee nearly touches the floor. Push yourself back up to the starting position. That's 1 repetition. Then repeat the move with the other leg.

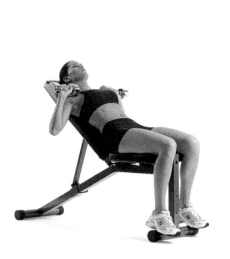
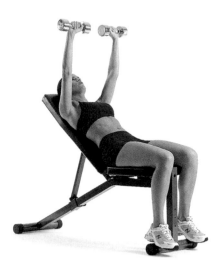

INCLINE PRESS

Grab a pair of dumbbells and lie on an incline bench, with your hips and thighs in a straight line and parallel to the floor. Press the weights straight up, then lower them to your chest, and repeat.

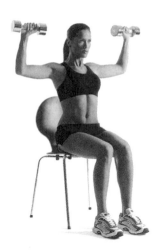 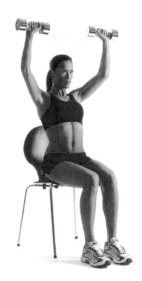

DUMBBELL PRESS

Sitting on an exercise bench, hold dumbbells at shoulder height. Press the weights straight overhead so that your arms are almost fully extended, hold for a count of one, then bring them down to the front of your shoulders. Repeat.

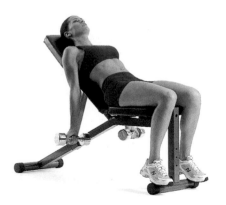 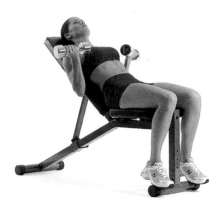

INCLINE DUMBBELL CURL

Lying back on an incline bench, hold the dumbbells with palms facing forward. Curl the weights up to your shoulders.

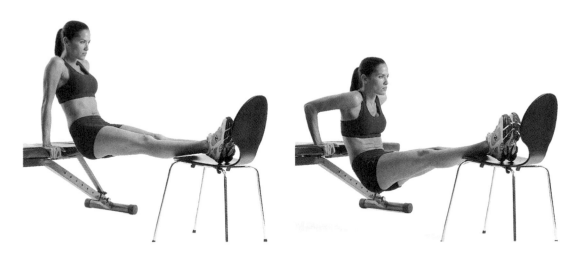

BENCH DIP

Stand with your back to a bench and place your hands on the edge, fingers pointing toward your lower back. Place your feet on a chair or another bench a few feet in front of you. Keeping your hands in place, slowly step forward until your legs are extended in front of you, knees slightly bent. Your arms ahould be straight, elbows unlocked, supporting your weight. Slowly bend your arms to lower yourself as far as you can and bring your butt as close to the floor as possible. Press yourself back up to the starting position. Do 10 to 12 repetitions.

"THANKS, ABS DIET!"

LOU HERNANDEZ

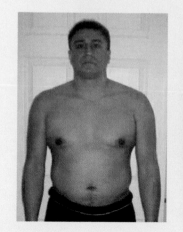 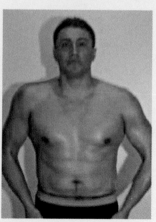

WEIGHT, WEEK 1: 211
WEIGHT, WEEK 6: 193

"Life had gotten me down after a divorce and the death of my father. After reading the diet, I knew the Abs Diet was the catalyst to get me back on track. I'm back to running 5Ks in record time, and I'm regaining my athletic physique. Not only do I have energy for my three kids, I've been able to change their bad eating habits. And most importantly, I've regained my confidence and outlook on life."

THE SWISS ARMY KNIFE WORKOUT: THE GREATEST ALL-IN-ONE MOVE

Whether it's duct tape or WD-40, most of us like anything that can serve lots of purposes. In that spirit, I recommend you try this one-move workout. Go through the move without any weight at first to get the sequence down, then add weight. Do 4 to 6 repetitions. Rest 2 minutes after every set. Try for 3 to 5 sets.

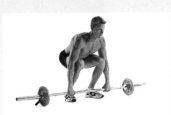

STEP 1

Squat over a barbell with your feet shoulder-width apart and your arms and back straight. TIP: You can also perform the move by holding a set of dumbbells instead.

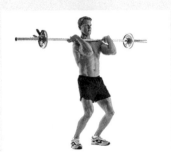

STEP 2

Stand up, shrug your shoulders, and, rising up on your toes, explosively pull the bar to chest level and "catch" it on your front shoulders by dropping under it into a partial squat, as you turn your elbows underneath the bar so your palms face up. Your upper arms should be parallel to the floor when the bar lands on your shoulders.

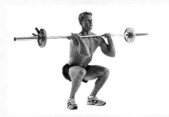

STEP 3

Lower your body into a full front squat—or at least until your thighs are parallel to the floor—by pushing your hips back and bending your knees as much as possible. Keep your back slightly arched in its natural alignment.

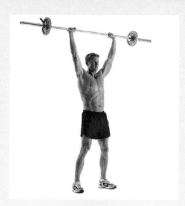

STEP 4

In one move, drive your feet into the floor and straighten your knees as you press the barbell over your head until your elbows lock.

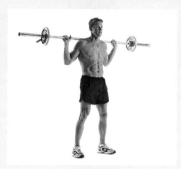

STEP 5

Pause, then lower the barbell behind your head and rest it on your upper back as you would when performing a squat.

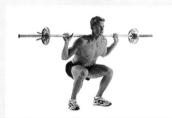

STEP 6

Lower your body into a full back squat—like the front squat, except for the position of the barbell.

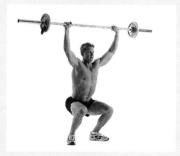

STEP 7

In one move, drive your feet into the floor and straighten your knees as you press the barbell over your head until your elbows lock. Pause, then return the barbell to the starting position.

The Have-a-Ball Workout: Go Round to Get Flat

One look at any gym in the country and you'll see that everyone is playing ball. That's because stability balls and medicine balls are exercise's version of a software upgrade—more tricks, more advantages, faster results. Stability balls keep you unbalanced during most moves—meaning that your core has to do extra work to keep you stabilized (so it's like an additional ab workout throughout your whole circuit). And the medicine ball—once the staple of the gray sweatsuit–wearing exercisers of the past—serves as a versatile form of resistance in various exercises. This circuit works at home or in the gym. All you need is a stability ball, a medicine ball, and a pair of dumbbells.

EXERCISE	REPETITIONS	REST	SETS
Swiss Ball Pushup	10–20	30 seconds	2
Leg Tuck	8–10	30 seconds	2
Swiss Ball Row Combination	10–12	30 seconds	2
Lateral Lunge	10 each side	30 seconds	2
Uneven Bench Press	6, switch sides	30 seconds	2
Jump Squat and Toss	10–12	30 seconds	2
Swiss Ball Prone Military Press	10–12	30 seconds	2
Hamstring Swiss Ball Curl	8–12	30 seconds	2
Swiss Ball Triceps Extension	12	30 seconds	2
Swiss Ball Curl	8–10 each arm	30 seconds	2

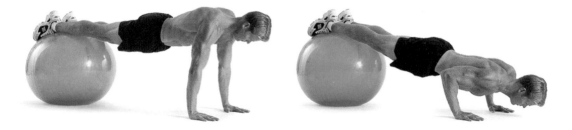

SWISS BALL PUSHUP

Get into a pushup position with your shins on a Swiss ball and your hands on the floor. Perform a traditional pushup by lowering your upper body toward the floor.

VARIATION 1: *Lift one leg off the ball and do half the number of your regular set. Change legs and do an equal number.*

VARIATION 2: *Move your hands out so they're 6 inches farther apart than normal.*

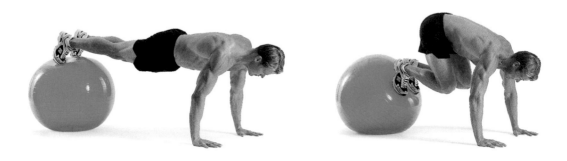

LEG TUCK

Start with your hands on the floor and your toes on a stability ball. Roll the ball toward you by bending your knees and pulling the ball with your feet. Pause, then roll the ball back to the starting position.

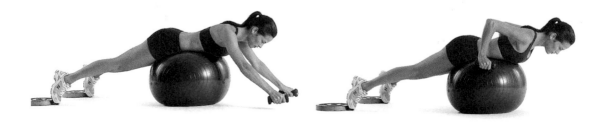

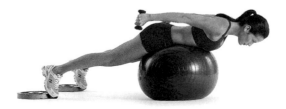

SWISS BALL ROW COMBINATION

Lie facedown on a Swiss ball and hold a pair of dumbbells (thumbs up) with your arms hanging down and forward at 45-degree angles to the floor. Pull the weights to your chest, then back to the sides of your butt. Return the weights to the starting position.

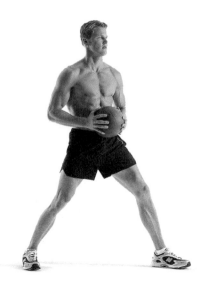
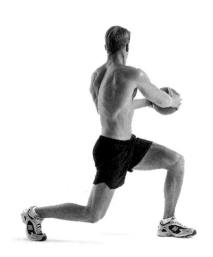

LATERAL LUNGE

Stand with your feet about 6 inches wider than hip width and hold a medicine ball in front of your belly. Lower your body by bending your left knee so your thigh is almost parallel to the floor, as you twist your torso and reach your arms to the left. Repeat on the other side.

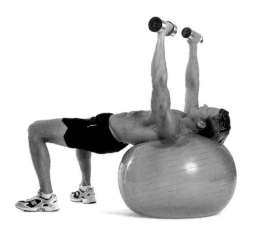
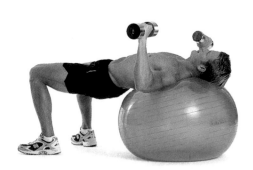

UNEVEN BENCH PRESS

Lie on a Swiss ball and hold dumbbells of different weights in each hand at chest level, palms facing away from you. Press the weights up and then lower them. Focus on keeping the heavier dumbbell from dipping lower than the lighter one. Do half the repetitions, then switch weights.

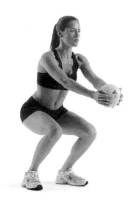

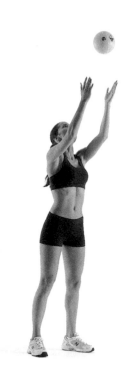

JUMP SQUAT AND TOSS

Grab a medicine ball and hold it with straight arms so it's in front of your belly button. Lower your body until your thighs are parallel to the floor. Pause, then jump up as you toss the ball into the air. Move to catch the ball, then get back into position and repeat.

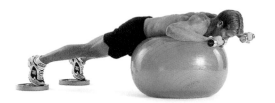 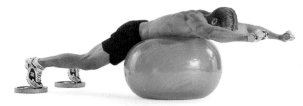

SWISS BALL PRONE MILITARY PRESS

Lie facedown on a stability ball and hold a pair of dumbbells at your shoulders, palms facing the floor. Press your arms straight out and forward so they're in line with your head. Pause, then return to the starting position.

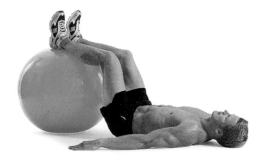 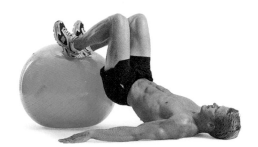

HAMSTRING SWISS BALL CURL

Lie on the floor with your heels and calves on top of a stability ball, your upper back and shoulders on the floor and your arms out to the sides. Raise your hips and your lower back off the ground so they form a straight line with your legs. Keeping your abs tight, pull the ball toward your butt by digging your heels into the ball until your feet are flat and your knees and butt are high in the air. Pause, then push the ball away from you until you legs are straight.

VARIATION: *Double the resistance by lifting one leg off the ball and pulling the ball with your other leg.*

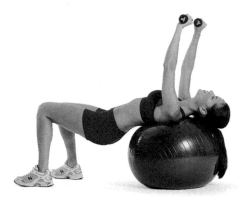 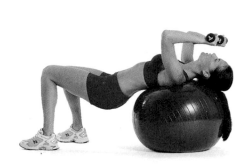

SWISS BALL TRICEPS EXTENSION

Grab a pair of dumbbells and sit on a stability ball. Roll your back down the ball, keeping your stomach tight, until your shoulders are pressed firmly against the ball and your butt is off the ball. Hold the weights with straight arms, angled so the weights are over your forehead. Keeping your upper arms still, bend at the elbows to lower the weights until they're even with the top of your forehead. Pause, then straighten your arms.

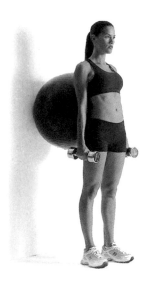 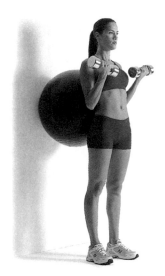

SWISS BALL BICEPS CURL

Place a Swiss ball against the wall a few feet up from the floor and stand with your lower back against the ball, holding it in place. Hold the dumbbells with palms facing the sides of your thighs. Curl the weights up, rotating your wrists upward so your palms face you by the time the weights reach your shoulders.

The Clean-Your-Plate Workout: Grab It, Move It, Work It

During crowded times at the gym—say, January 2, or 6 weeks before beach season—it's harder to find an unused piece of equipment than it is to hail a cab at 5 o'clock on a rainy Friday in New York. No worries. You can get a great full-body workout by using something that every gym has plenty of—weight plates. Claim a bench and a few plates of different weights, and you'll have all the equipment you need to do this circuit.

EXERCISE	REPETITIONS	REST	SETS
Bench Press Pullover	10	30 seconds	2
Bear-Hug Front Lunge	10–15 each leg	30 seconds	2
Hammer Curl	10	30 seconds	2
Non-Lock Squat	15	30 seconds	2
Single-Arm Bentover Row	10 each arm	30 seconds	2
Stiff-Legged Deadlift Curl and Press	10	30 seconds	2
Front Raise Rotation	10	30 seconds	2

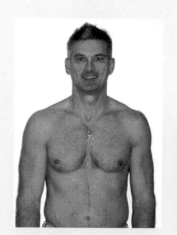
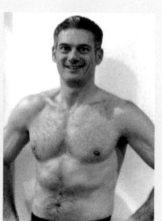

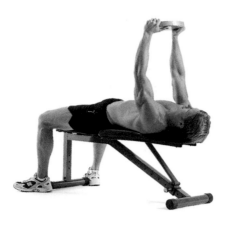
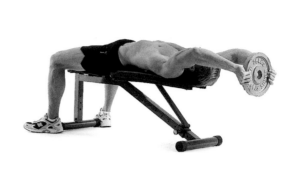

BENCH PRESS PULLOVER

Lie faceup on a bench and grasp the sides of the weight plate. Press the weight to arms' length. Keep your arms extended and lower the weight behind your head until it's in line with your body. Raise it above your head again, then lower it back to your chest.

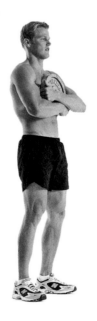
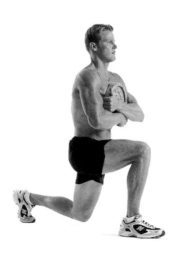

BEAR-HUG FRONT LUNGE

Standing, hold the plate across your chest. Lunge a step forward until your front shin is perpendicular to the floor and your thigh is parallel to it. Keep your torso upright, and return to the starting position. Switch legs.

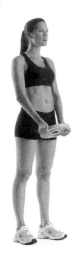 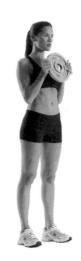

HAMMER CURL

Grab the weight plate with both hands and hold it in front of your thighs. Curl it up toward your face until the top of the plate is under your chin, then return.

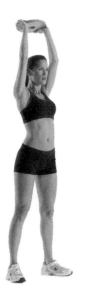 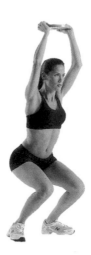

NON-LOCK SQUAT

Hold the plate above your head with elbows locked, and squat deeply, until your thighs are parallel to the ground. Keep your knees slightly flexed, and don't pause at the top of the movement.

VARIATION: *Hold the plate in a bear hug in front of your torso to rest your upper body during this exercise.*

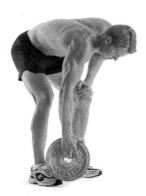 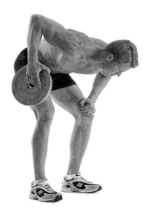

SINGLE-ARM BENT-OVER ROW

Hold the plate through the hole with the middle three fingers of your right hand. Bend over and rest your left hand on your thigh. Pull the plate to your shoulder. As you do, squeeze your shoulders blade toward the middle of your back. Do a set, then switch arms.

"THANKS, ABS DIET!"

BRIAN WUBBEN

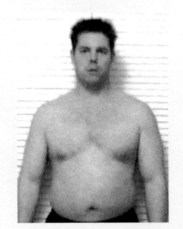 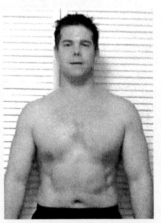

WEIGHT, WEEK 1: 215
WEIGHT, WEEK 6: 195

"The Abs Diet is so much more than just an eating plan. It's helped me to see how working out and nutrition go together to get results. I've lifted weights off and on, but I've never really gotten much to show for it, so I didn't stick to anything long-term. This plan is one I can see myself sticking to for a long time."

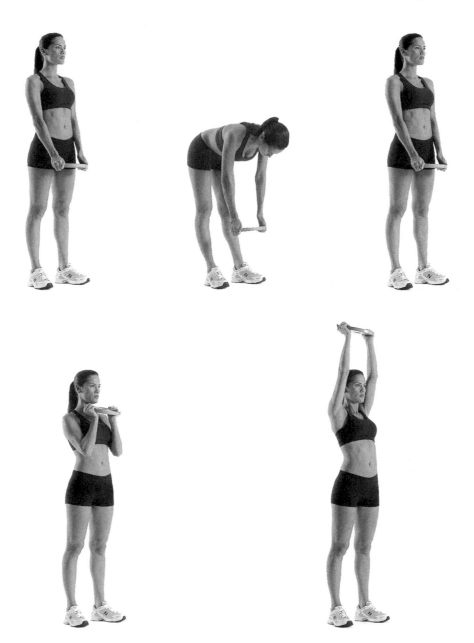

STIFF-LEGGED DEADLIFT CURL AND PRESS

Hold the weight at waist level, with your knees slightly bent. Lower the weight by bending from your waist; keep your back straight. Return to the starting position. Curl the weight to your chest, then press it above your head. Finish in the starting position.

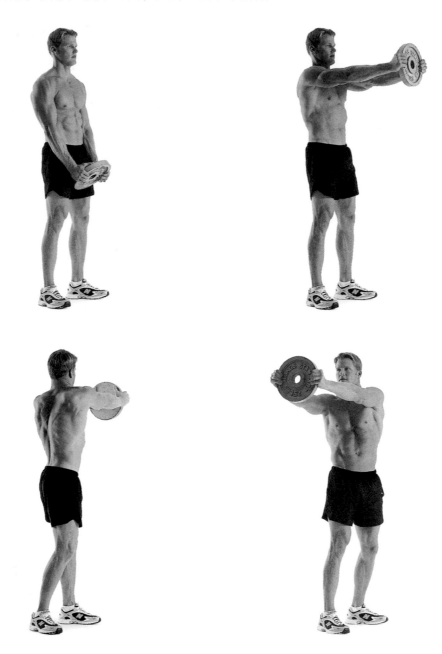

FRONT RAISE ROTATION

From a standing position, lift the weight to eye level with your arms extended straight out in front of you. Slowly turn your head and torso 90 degrees to the left. Reverse the movement and twist 180 degrees to the right. Turn back so you're facing straight ahead again.

The Band-Aid Workout: Stretch for Strength

Since carry-on bags now seem smaller than Ziplocs (and many hotel gyms are smaller than closets), it's not always easy to exercise on the road. Still, you can get a perfectly good workout with minimal investment by using exercise bands. Hook them onto chairs and doorknobs and you create tension that provides the resistance you need for a strength workout. Pack the bands, and do this circuit in your hotel room.

EXERCISE	REPETITIONS	REST	SETS
Band Lunge	10–15	30 seconds	3
Band Standing Row	10–12	30 seconds	3
Romanian Deadlift	10–12	30 seconds	3
Band Standing Chest Press	10–12	30 seconds	3
Reverse Woodchop	10–15 each side	30 seconds	3
Overhead Crunch	15	30 seconds	3

"THANKS, ABS DIET!"

NATHAN KITTS

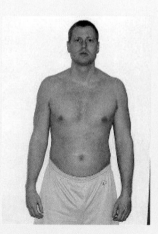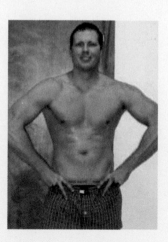

WEIGHT, WEEK 1: 212
WEIGHT, WEEK 6: 195

"For the first week of the Abs Diet I thought it wasn't going to work. I just wasn't hungry enough. By the end of the program I knew I was wrong. I have lost fat while gaining muscle definition and strength. My blood pressure has dropped 10 points, lowering my dependence on medicine. I intend to adopt the Abs Diet as a lifestyle, rather than a diet program, for the rest of my life."

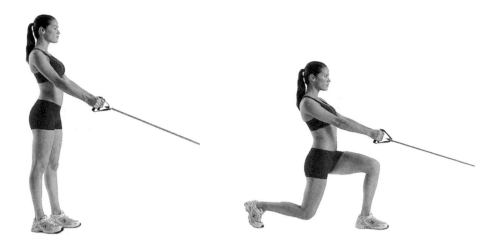

BAND LUNGE

Connect the band near the floor and grab a handle with each hand. Step forward with your non-dominant leg and lower your body until your front knee is bent 90 degrees and your other knee nearly touches the floor. Push yourself back up to the starting position as quickly as you can. That's 1 repetition. Repeat the move with the other leg.

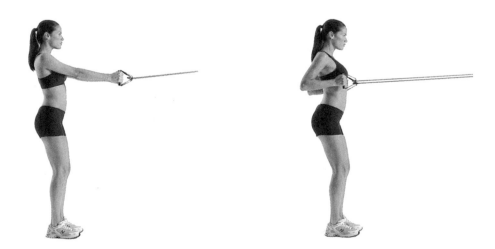

BAND STANDING ROW

Connect the band at the level of your chest and grab a handle with each hand, palms facing each other. Stand with your feet shoulder-width apart and your knees slightly bent. Squeeze your shoulder blades together and pull the handles to your chest until your elbows are bent at a 90-degree angle. Return to the starting position and repeat.

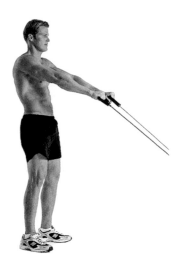
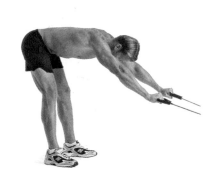

ROMANIAN DEADLIFT

Connect the band near the floor and grab a handle with each hand, palms facing the floor. Stand with your feet shoulder-width apart and your knees slightly bent. Bend at your hips (keep your back flat) and lower your upper body as far as possible or until it's parallel to the floor. Pause, then pull your torso back up to the starting position and repeat.

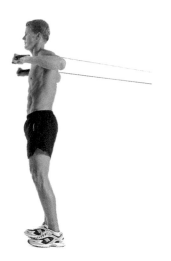
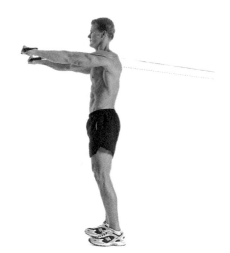

BAND STANDING CHEST PRESS

Connect the band at the level of your chest and turn around and face the opposite direction. Grab a handle with each hand and hold them next to the sides of your chest. Push the handles out in front of you until your arms are extended. Return to the starting position and repeat.

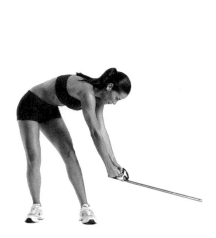
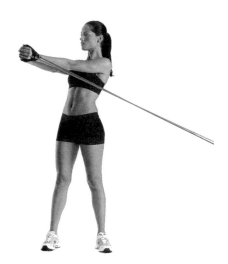

REVERSE WOOD CHOP

Connect the band near the floor and hold the handles together in both hands. Stand with your left side toward the band connection. Bend over and hold the handles just outside your left calf. Pull the handles up and across your torso as you twist your shoulders to the right. Return to the starting position. Finish the repetitions, then switch sides.

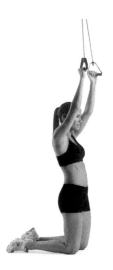
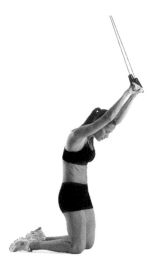

OVERHEAD CRUNCH

Connect the band above your head and grab a handle with each hand. Stand upright (or kneel) with your feet (or knees, if you have to kneel to do the exercise) shoulder-width apart and your arms straight but not locked. Without bending your arms, crunch your chest toward your pelvis. Pause, then return to the starting position and repeat.

The Body-Blaster Workout: Advanced Moves for an Advanced Body

If your body is harder than ancient Swiss cheese, then maybe you need exercises that will kick your caboose and take your fitness to the next level. This circuit utilizes exercises that will challenge your body in weight, in form, and in stability. And that's why I'm giving you a few extra seconds of rest in between each one. Grab your towel. You're going to sweat like a cold bottle of Bud at the edge of a Florida pool.

EXERCISE	REPETITIONS	REST	SETS
Double Swiss Ball Pushup	10	1 minute	2–3
Box Lunge	6–10 each side	1 minute	2–3
One–Arm Pulldown	5 each side	1 minute	2–3
Sumo Deadlift	10–12	1 minute	2–3
Gator Pushup	5 up, 5 back	1 minute	2–3
EZ-Curl Biceps Challenge	55	1 minute	2–3
Kneeling Hamstring Curl	2–10	1 minute	2–3

"THANKS, ABS DIET!"

LUKE VAN CAMP

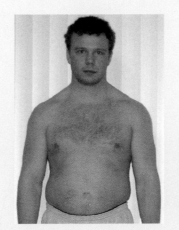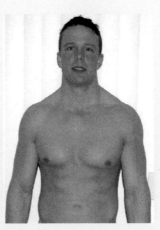

WEIGHT, WEEK 1: 210
WEIGHT, WEEK 6: 190

"I graduated high school at 145 pounds; ever since then I have been steadily gaining weight. I had tried various other diets, but I didn't stick to them and found myself having to upsize my wardrobe. The Abs Diet was a revelation to me. I lost 3 inches in my waist and 20 pounds! And unlike with other diets, I had plenty to eat, enjoyed the meals, and actually got stronger! This is something I'm sticking with."

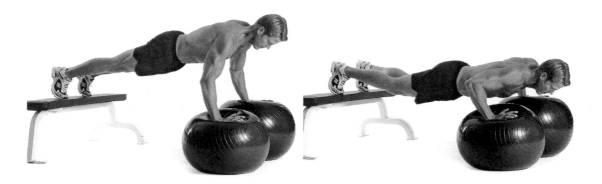

DOUBLE SWISS BALL PUSHUP

Set two Swiss balls a few feet in front of a bench. Place a hand on the center of each ball, making sure the balls are touching, and rest your feet on the bench. Lower your body as far as you can with control. Pause, then push yourself back up to the starting position. TIP: If this exercise is too difficult at first, have a partner stabilize the balls for you or lean them against a wall to brace them.

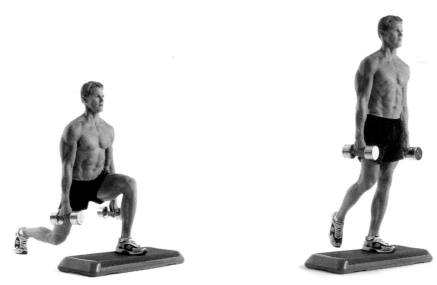

BOX LUNGE

Place an exercise step in front of you, stand with your feet hip-width apart, and hold two weights at your sides. Step forward onto the step with your left leg so that your left thigh ends up parallel to the floor and your knee is over your toes. Raise up onto the step, then step down and repeat to the other side.

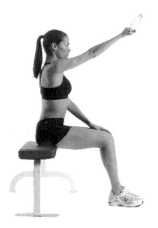
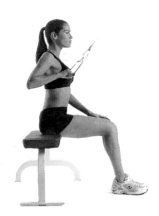

ONE-ARM PULLDOWN

Attach a single handle to a high-cable pulley. Sit on the seat with your feet flat on the floor and your back straight. Grasp the handle with your right hand, palm facing forward. Slowly pull the handle straight down until your forearm touches your side. Do not twist your back or arms during the pull. Return to the starting position in one smooth motion.

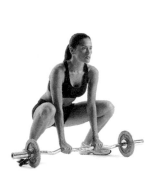
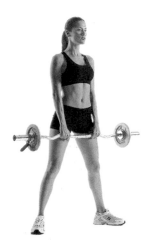

SUMO DEADLIFT

Squat behind a barbell with your feet wider than shoulder width and your toes pointed out at about 45 degrees. With your hands inside your knees, shoulders over the bar, and arms and back straight, grab the bar overhand. Push with your heels and stand up, keeping the bar in contact with your body. Finish standing upright with your shoulder blades back and down and your lower back flat. Pause, then slowly lower the weight back to the floor.

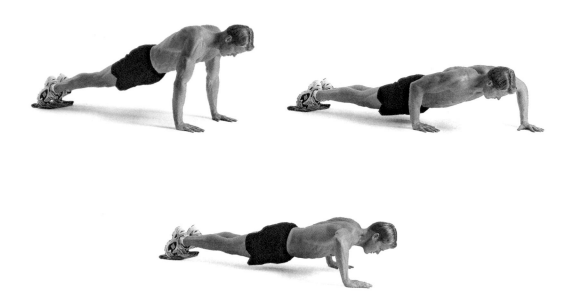

GATOR PUSHUP

Stand on a small towel and get into the classic pushup position, with your knees flexed and your hands directly under your shoulders. With your abs tight, walk your left hand out about a foot in front of your right hand and do a pushup. Now walk your right hand out about a foot in front of your left hand, drag your feet forward, and do another. Repeat this sequence five times, then reverse the move to walk back to the starting position.

ABS FACT

5 and 5

Number of seconds The Rock takes
to raise a weight, and then to lower it

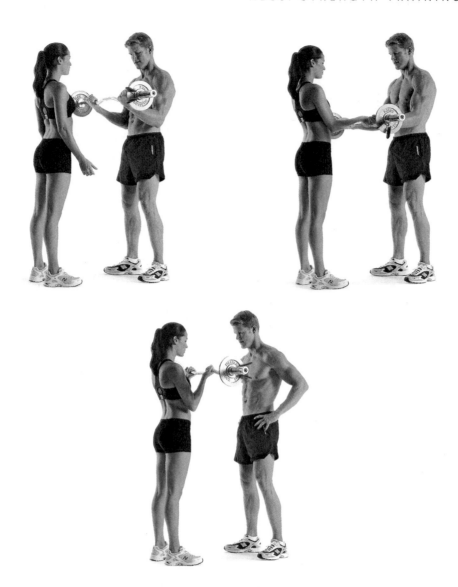

EZ-CURL BICEPS CHALLENGE

Set up an EZ-curl bar or barbell with a weight that challenges you and your training partner. Face your partner and perform a set of 10 curls in a 3–0–1 tempo (3 seconds down, no rest, 1 second up). Then, instead of setting the bar down, hand it to your partner so he or she can do 10 reps. Hand it back and forth for 9 repetitions, then 8, and so on. Work your way down until you've each done a single repetition with the bar.

VARIATION: *If you don't have a partner, rest the weight on the floor for 15 seconds in between sets.*

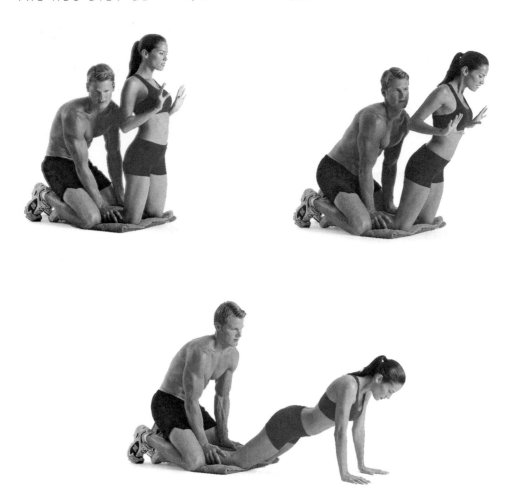

KNEELING HAMSTRING CURL

Kneel on a folded towel or an exercise mat. Keep your hands in front of your chest. Have a partner sit behind you, facing your back, pressing down on your lower legs with his hands. Keep your abs tight, chest up, and hips forward so your body forms a straight line from your ears to your knees. Maintain this posture as you lower your torso toward the floor while resisting gravity with your hamstrings and calves. Control the range of motion as far as you can, catch yourself with your hands, then push off the floor to assist your hamstrings and glutes in pulling you back up to the starting position.

VARIATION: *Once you've mastered the move, add weight by holding a weight plate close to your chest.*

The Hard-Core Hard-Core Workout: Moves for Every Muscle

Back for more? Going for a 24-pack? Okay, let's go at it again. Here's an alternative circuit for advanced lifters. Still not enough? Then combine Advanced Circuits 1 and 2, funny guy.

EXERCISE	REPETITIONS	REST	SETS
Barbell Pushup	10–12	1 minute	2–3
Reverse Lunge and Ball Twist	12–15 each side	1 minute	2–3
Uneven–Grip Pullup	4–6, each side	1 minute	2–3
Ball Catch and Straddle Jump	3	1 minute	2–3
Plyometric Pushup	8–12	1 minute	2–3
One and Quarter Squat	6	1 minute	2–3

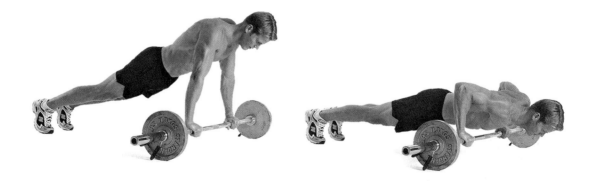

BARBELL PUSHUP

Get into the classic pushup position with your hands on a barbell (the kind that can roll away). Perform the classic pushup, but keep steady so the bar doesn't roll.

VARIATION: *Lift one leg off the floor and put it on top of the foot that's on the floor.*

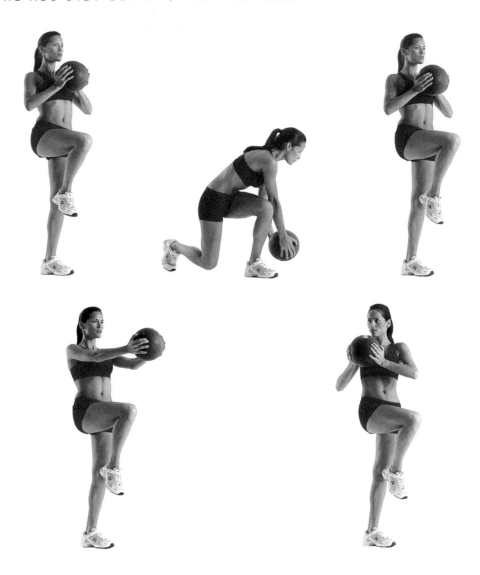

REVERSE LUNGE AND BALL TWIST

Stand holding a medicine ball in front of your chest with both hands. Step backward with your right leg and lower your body until your left knee is bent 90 degrees and your right knee nearly touches the floor (in a backward lunge position). Your left lower leg should be perpendicular to the floor. Twist to your left and touch the ball to the floor by leaning over your thigh and straightening your arms. Transfer your body weight to your left leg and push yourself to a standing position as you lift your right knee to your chest. Keeping the knee up, push the ball away from your chest, pull it back quickly, then twist your torso as far as you can to the right. Return to the starting position and repeat 14 times, then switch sides.

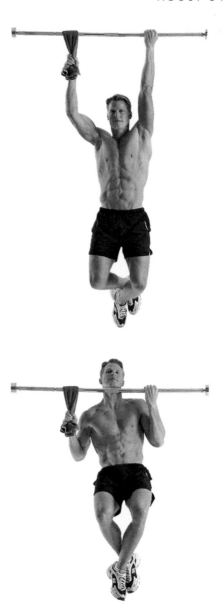

UNEVEN-GRIP PULLUP

Loop a towel over a pullup bar and hold both ends with your right hand. Grasp the bar with your left hand using an underhand grip. The vertical separation between your hands increases intensity on the higher arm. Pull up with both hands. TIP: If you have a hard time pulling yourself up, use a step or have a partner help you pull yourself up to the bar, then lower yourself down as slowly as possible.

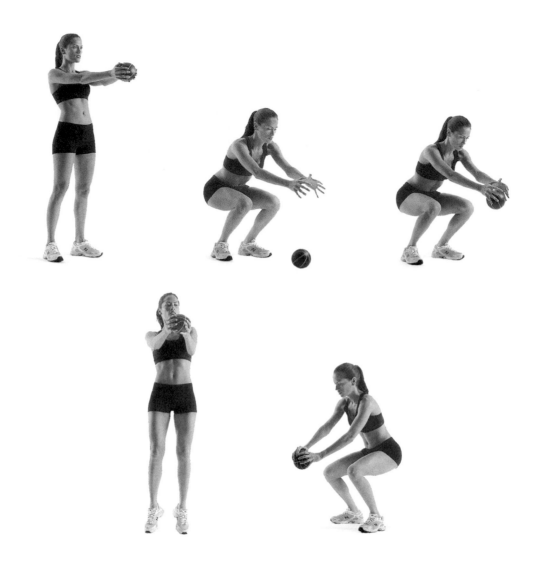

BALL CATCH AND STRADDLE JUMP

Stand holding a fitness ball in front of your chest with both hands, your feet shoulder-width apart. Drop the ball, then lower your body into a squat position and catch it after one bounce. As you catch the ball, immediately jump as high as you can and rotate your body 90 degrees to your right. When your feet touch the floor, bounce the ball, squat, and jump to the starting position. Repeat this to the left, and return to the starting position.

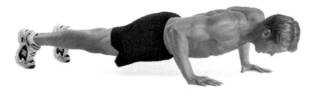

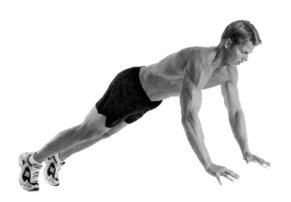

PLYOMETRIC PUSHUP

Set up in the classic pushup position on a well-padded carpet or exercise mat. Push up hard enough for your hands to come off the floor and catch some air. When you hit the floor, go immediately into the next repetition, pushing up again as hard as you can and catching more air.

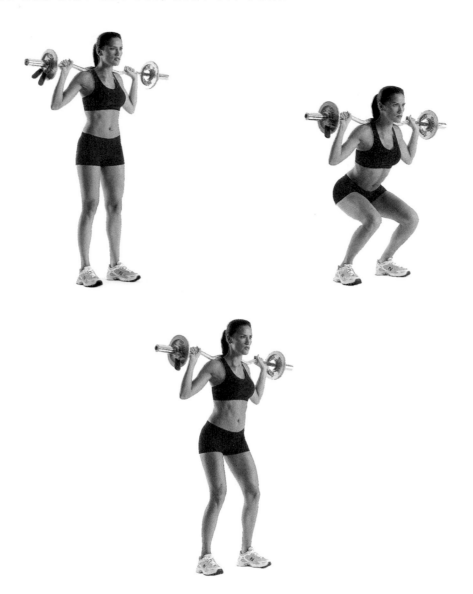

ONE-AND-A-QUARTER SQUAT

Load a barbell with as much weight as you can squat six times and stand with the bar on your shoulders. Squat until your thighs are parallel to the floor, pause, then push your body up until your knees are a quarter of the way back to vertical. Pause, then lower your body back down. Pause, then push back to the starting position. That's 1 repetition.

The Workout Buffet: Choose Your Own Moves

What I like most about the ABS3 approach is that there are virtually limitless ways to add lean muscle mass. As long as you follow the major principles, you will continually challenge your body—which will make it grow—and shrink—in the way that you want. That's why I want to give you a list of exercise ingredients, so you can come up with your own recipes for strength-training circuits. I've broken it down by muscle groups and included many multi-muscle moves. For all exercises, aim for 10 to 12 repetitions, unless otherwise noted. And then construct your own plan. This is the plan I'd suggest:

Option 1: Pick three to five multi-muscle moves and perform them in a circuit, with no more than 30 seconds between exercises. After you finish the circuit, rest for 2 minutes, then repeat. For programs with three moves, do the circuit three to five times. For programs with five moves, do it two or three times.

Option 2: Construct a program based on exercises that emphasize different muscle groups. Pick one from each category as follows and perform in a circuit—twice through for beginners, three times for intermediate and advanced. Follow this circuit:

1. Leg exercise

2. Chest exercise

3. Back exercise

4. Leg exercise

5. Shoulder exercise

6. Leg exercise

7. Biceps exercise

8. Triceps exercise

9. Leg exercise

Option 3: Pick one leg-oriented multi-muscle move to start and end the circuit, and add in one move each from the biggest-muscle groups (chest, back, shoulders, and legs). Follow this circuit:

1. Multi-muscle exercise that includes a lunge or squat

2. Chest exercise

3. Leg exercise

4. Back exercise

5. Shoulder exercise

6. Multi-muscle exercise that includes a lunge or squat

MULTI-MUSCLES

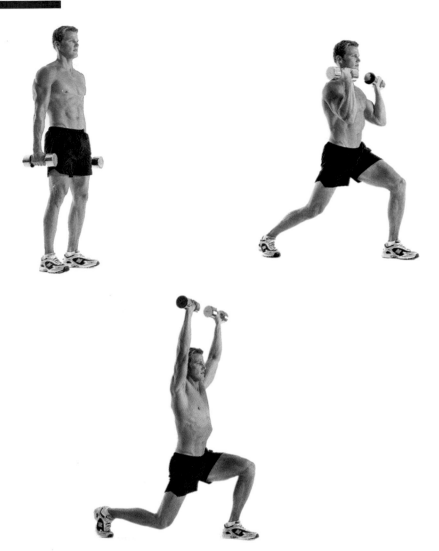

LUNGING CURL TO PRESS

Stand holding a pair of dumbbells at your sides, palms toward you. As you begin to curl the weights up to your shoulders, take a large step forward with your left foot; your hands should reach shoulder height by the time your foot is planted. As soon as the weights reach your shoulders, press them overhead while you lower your body until your left thigh is parallel to the floor. Fully extend your arms by the time your thigh is level. Return to the starting position, and repeat with your right leg. That's 1 repetition. Do 8 to 12 on each leg.

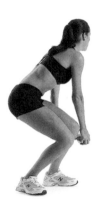
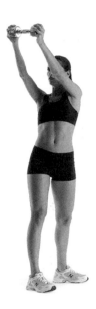

CORKSCREW

Begin in a squat position—thighs parallel to the floor—holding a dumbbell with both hands at arm's length to the outside of your left ankle. As you push yourself up to a standing position, keep your arms extended and rotate your torso to bring the dumbbell above your opposite ear. Then lower the weight and your body back to the starting position. That's 1 repetition. Repeat on the other side. Do 8 to 10 repetitions.

"THANKS, ABS DIET!"

JEREMY KOPPUS

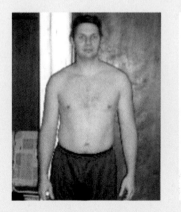
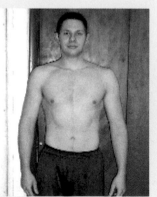

WEIGHT, WEEK 1: 179
WEIGHT, WEEK 6: 167

"You do not have to sacrifice taste and good food to lose weight. By taking the challenge I have lost weight, I can now take the stairs without getting winded, I avoid the elevators, my asthma has improved, and I feel great. My mid-section is stronger and leaner than ever!"

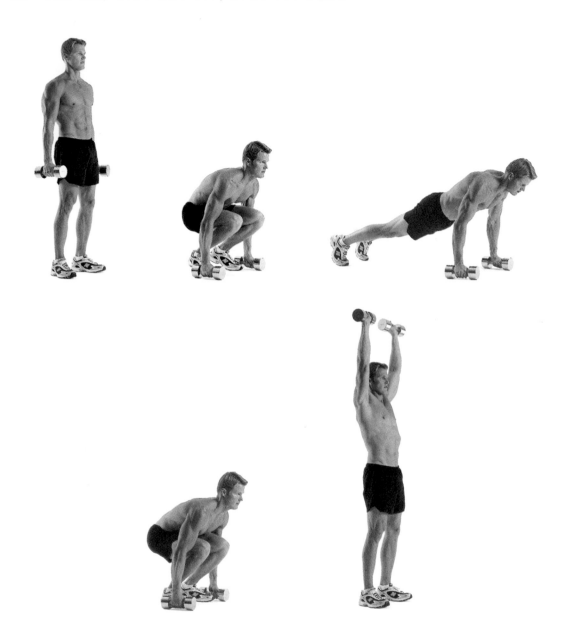

DUMBBELL SQUAT THRUST AND PRESS

Stand holding a pair of light dumbbells at arm's length at your sides. Lower your body quickly, touching the dumbbells to the floor, then kick your legs out behind you so you're in the classic pushup position. Now bring your legs forward again so your feet are under your shoulders, stand up, and press the weights overhead. Return to the starting position. Do 10 to 12 repetitions.

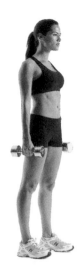

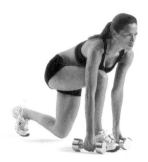

LUNGE AND TOUCH

Stand holding a pair of dumbbells at your sides. Keeping your feet pointed forward and your abs braced tight, step forward with one foot, lower your body so that your forward thigh is parallel to the floor and your rear thigh is perpendicular to the floor, and reach the floor with your arms on opposite sides of the lunging knee. Touch the dumbbells to the floor, then push back to the starting position. Do 5 or 6 repetitions. (Lunge to the left and right to complete 1 repetition.)

"THANKS, ABS DIET!"

ROBERT WOODSON

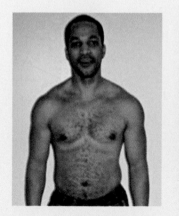 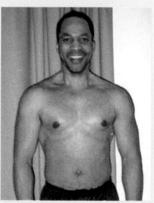

WEIGHT, WEEK 1: 182
WEIGHT, WEEK 6: 170

"Not only do I feel great and have lots more energy, it has provided a great new lifestyle. While going through a divorce I needed a distraction and going to the gym was my outlet. I was just throwing weights around until I found the *Abs Diet* book. This was the first time I have ever been on a plan, and it was great."

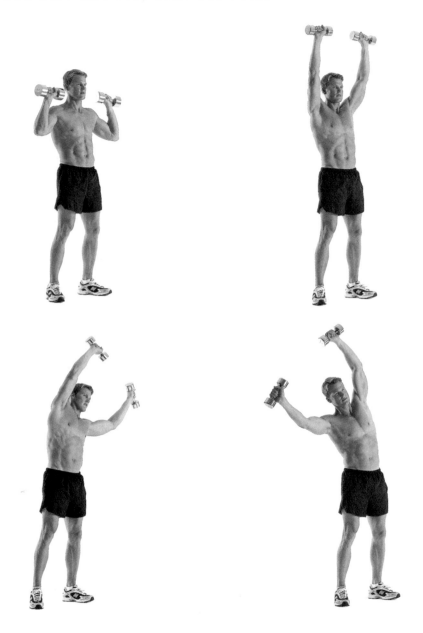

SHOULDER PRESS WITH SAXON SIDE BEND

Hold a pair of light dumbbells at your shoulders. Press the weights overhead. Keeping your knees flexed and your abs tight, bend at the waist to the left. Return to the center, using your abs to straighten up. Lower the weights to your shoulders and repeat, this time bending to the right. Do 8 to 10 repetitions.

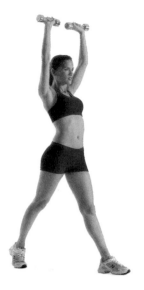 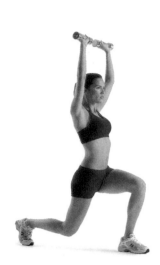

OVERHEAD SPLIT SQUAT

Grab a light pair of dumbbells and step one foot 2 to 3 feet in front of the other. Rise onto the ball of your back foot and lift the weights over your head. Now bend both knees and lower your body until your back knee almost touches the floor and your front knee forms a 90-degree angle. Keeping your arms straight, push yourself back up to the starting position. Do 5 or 6 repetitions on each foot.

"THANKS, ABS DIET!"

JOHN SMITH

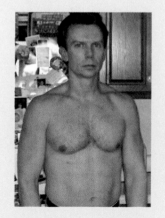 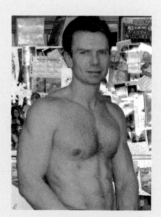

WEIGHT, WEEK 1: 166
WEIGHT, WEEK 6: 158

"I've worked out all my adult life, with the goal of obtaining a 6-pack. Little did I know I was going about it the wrong way. I rarely ate breakfast, worked my abs virtually every day, hardly ever worked my legs, and never did aerobic exercise. Thanks to the Abs Diet, at the age of 43, I eat better, exercise less, and have the abs I've never had before."

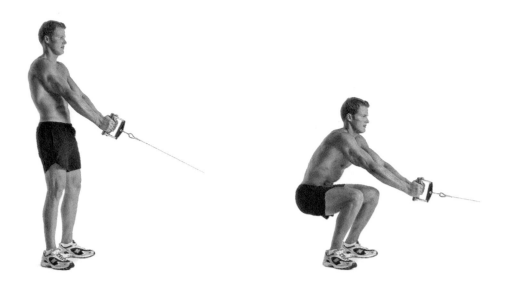

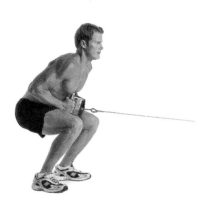

SQUAT TO ROW

Attach universal grips (straps with handles) to the low pulley of a cable station. Facing the weight stack, grab the handles with a neutral grip (palms facing each other) and take a few steps back. With your arms straight, squat until your thighs are at least parallel to the floor; keep your knees from going in front of your toes. Pull the handles to the bottom of your rib cage, keeping your elbows in and squeezing your shoulder blades together. Pause, extend your arms so that they're straight once again, then return to the starting position.

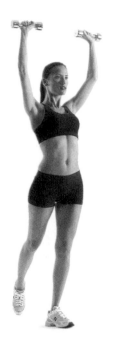

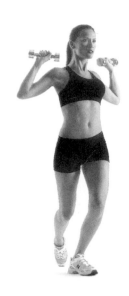

ONE-LEG SQUAT PRESS

Stand on your left leg and lift your right leg in the air behind your left, extending it to the left as far as possible. Hold a pair of light dumbbells above your head. Lower yourself in a one-legged squat until your right foot touches the ground. As you go down, lower the weights. Lift the weights over your head as you return to standing. Do 20 to 30 repetitions on each leg.

VARIATION: *Do the exercise on a step, increase the weights, or try standing on something slightly unstable—like a pillow, foam roller, or balance board.*

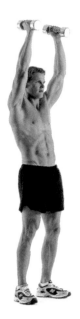

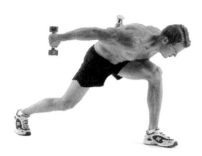

STRIKING REVERSE LUNGE

Grab a pair of light dumbbells and hold them above your shoulders at arm's length as you stand with your feet shoulder-width apart. Begin by striding back with one leg into a reverse-lunge position as you simultaneously thrust your arms down and back behind you. In the bottom position, your arms will be straight behind you and your torso will be facedown over your front thigh. Pause for a second, then push down with the heel of your front foot as you return to the starting position, simultaneously thrusting your arms overhead. Repeat with the opposite leg leading back into the reverse lunge. That's 1 repetition. Do 8 on each side.

"THANKS, ABS DIET!"

BYRON MARKUS

WEIGHT, WEEK 1: 210
WEIGHT, WEEK 6: 199

"I have learned good health should not be taken for granted. Just weeks before I started the 6-week challenge, I found out my dad had cancer. My dad had always been healthy and ac-

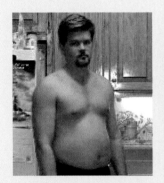

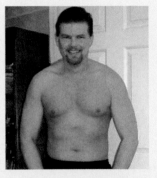

tive prior to this. I could not have stuck to the diet and continued it without the help of my wife making my meals and my little boy always telling me I could succeed."

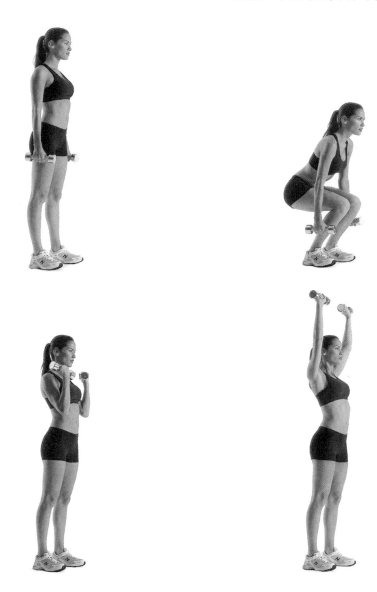

SQUAT TO CURL TO PRESS

Stand holding a pair of dumbbells at your sides, palms facing in. Lower your body until your thighs are parallel to the floor. Pause, then push yourself back up as you curl the weights up to your shoulders, rotating your wrists toward you as they rise. Now rotate your wrists away from you as you press the weights above your head, so your palms face forward at the top of the move. Then lower the weights to your shoulders, and finally back to the starting position. Do 8 to 12 repetitions.

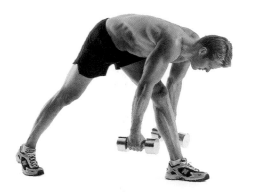
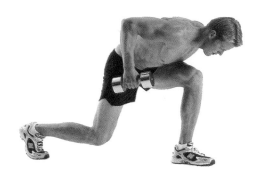

STATIONARY LUNGE AND ROW

Stand holding a pair of dumbbells at your sides, palms facing in. Step straight back with one foot, allowing only the ball of that foot to touch the floor behind you. Bend forward at the hips until your torso is almost parallel to the floor; that's the starting position. As you pull the weights up to your rib cage, lower your body until your back knee is 2 to 3 inches above the floor. Your front knee should be over your toes. Lower the weights as you push yourself back up to the starting position.

"THANKS, ABS DIET!"

CARL GEOPPINGER

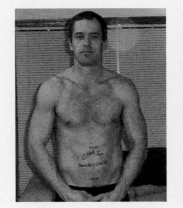
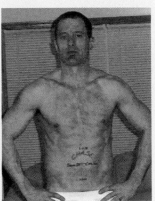

WEIGHT, WEEK 1: 162
WEIGHT, WEEK 6: 148

"The Abs Diet has taught me to eat more sensibly and learn about proper nutrition and exercise, and given me more energy. It has also helped me to be a happier person. I like the way I look. I enjoy doing the workouts, and most of all I love the way I feel after I'm through working out. But the biggest thing that it has done for me is help me to live a healthier lifestyle."

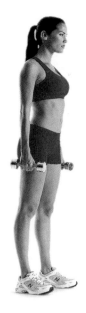
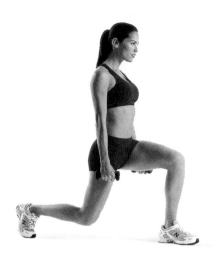
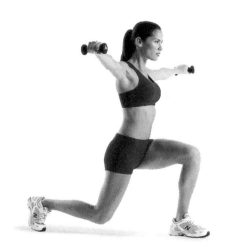

LUNGE WITH LATERAL RAISE

Stand holding a pair of light dumbbells at your sides, palms facing in. Take a large step forward with your left leg, until your right knee is close to the floor. (Don't allow your left knee to go beyond your toes.) Now raise the dumbbells up and out to the sides until your arms are parallel to the floor. Pause, then lower the dumbbells under control as you push yourself back up to the starting position. Finish a set of 10, then switch legs and repeat.

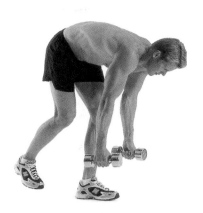
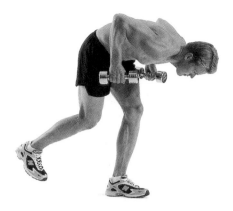

SINGLE-LEG BENT-OVER ROW

Stand holding a pair of light dumbbells in front of you with a parallel grip (palms facing each other). Raise one leg slightly off the floor and bend the other slightly. Bend forward at the hips until your torso is almost parallel to the floor. Let your arms hang down so the weights are near your ankles. Pull the weights up to the sides of your chest, squeezing your shoulder blades together at the top of the move. Pause, then return to the starting position. Stand on the opposite leg for the second set.

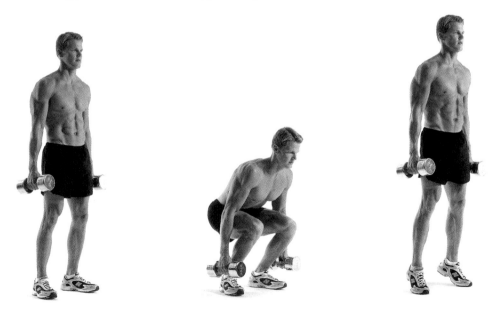

SQUAT AND CALF RAISE

Stand holding a pair of dumbbells with your arms straight, palms facing toward your thighs. Slowly squat down until your thighs are almost parallel to the floor, then push yourself back up into a standing position. At the top of the move, rise up onto the balls of your feet so that your heels lift off the floor as far as possible. Drop your heels back down to the floor and repeat the move.

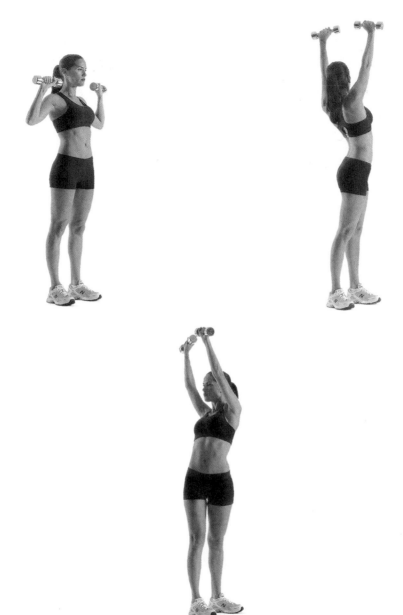

TWISTING SHOULDER PRESS

Hold a pair of dumbbells outside your shoulders at jaw level, palms facing forward. Press the dumbbells overhead as you twist your torso to the left. Lower the dumbbells as you twist back to center, then press upward again while twisting to the right. Do 6 repetitions in each direction.

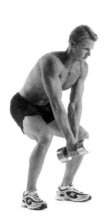
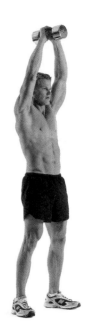

DUMBBELL SWING

Stand holding a dumbbell with a hand-over-hand grip at arms' length in front of your waist. Bend at your knees and waist (keep your back flat) until your upper body is about 45 degrees from vertical and the dumbbell is between your knees. Swing the dumbbell up and directly over your head (as if you were raising an ax) as you straighten your knees and back and push your hips forward. Pause, then lower the dumbbell back to the starting position and repeat. Do 8 repetitions.

"THANKS, ABS DIET!"

DONALD LATIMER

WEIGHT, WEEK 1: 165
WEIGHT, WEEK 6: 155

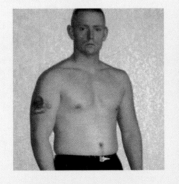
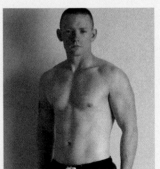

"I'm a United States Marine. I have always been able to play the part of the perfect Marine, yet no matter what I tried, I have never been able to look the part. I was always able to gain muscle but never able to slim my midsection. This program has helped me become the ideal Marine. Now I not only have good leadership qualities, but I'm in the best shape that I have ever been."

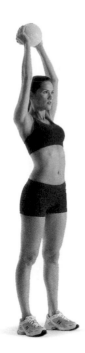
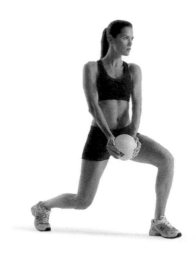

OVERHEAD LUNGE

Hold a medicine ball at arm's length over your head, your feet hip-width apart and your knees slightly bent. Step forward with your left foot and lower your body so that your left lower leg is perpendicular to the floor and your left thigh is parallel to the floor. At the same time, keep your arms straight and lower the medicine ball to your right until it's even with your left thigh. Return to the starting position by pushing off your left leg and raising the medicine all back over your head. Repeat, stepping forward with your right leg. Do a total of 12 repetitions, 6 for each leg, alternating legs each time.

"I WASN'T IN THIS GOOD A SHAPE IN THE NAVY"

Name: John Hanson

Age: 35

Height: 5'6"

Starting weight: 175

Six weeks later: 160

Starting waist size: 34"

Six weeks later: 32"

John Hanson has tried hundreds of different exercise programs but none of them seemed to work. When he tried the Abs Diet, it became the little buddy that pushed him along. What was most amazing? How easy it was.

"Right off the bat, I had increased energy," he says. "Even with three kids and how busy I was, it was really easy. It just took a few days for things like the sugar cravings to go away. But it was a really easy diet."

A self-proclaimed meat-and-potatoes guy, Hanson easily adjusted to the Power 12 foods and now is trying to get his kids eating them, too. Hanson's biggest revelation came from looking at labels—and seeing all the foods with fat-inducing high-fructose corn syrup and trans fats in them.

The plan has not only given him more energy but also made him more productive at work. "I work for a non-profit and wear six different hats, and I have more focus at work," he says. "The six weeks went really quick. It's really exciting to see the results of before and after. I can't believe I'm the same guy. At 35, I'm in better shape than when I was in the Navy and running 5 and 6 miles every day and exercising every day. It's crazy."

LEGS

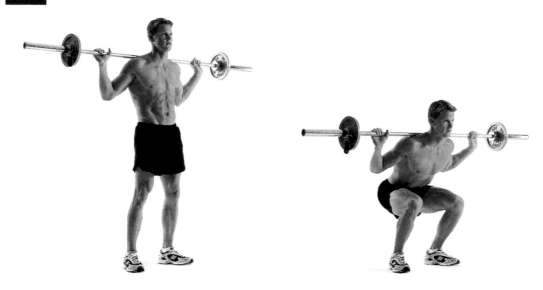

PAUSE SQUAT

Hold a barbell across your shoulders and lower your body until your thighs are parallel to the ground. Pause for 4 seconds, then push your body back up to the starting position. Do 10 repetitions.

"THANKS, ABS DIET!"

RAYMOND JAMES

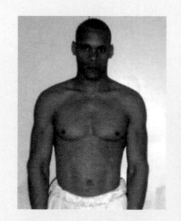 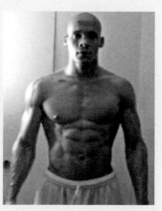

WEIGHT, WEEK 1: 165
WEIGHT, WEEK 6: 150

"I maintained strength, gained speed and flexibility, all the while establishing power through a new range of motion. I know now that the knowledge obtained is far greater than any prize that could be gained, and for that I am thankful."

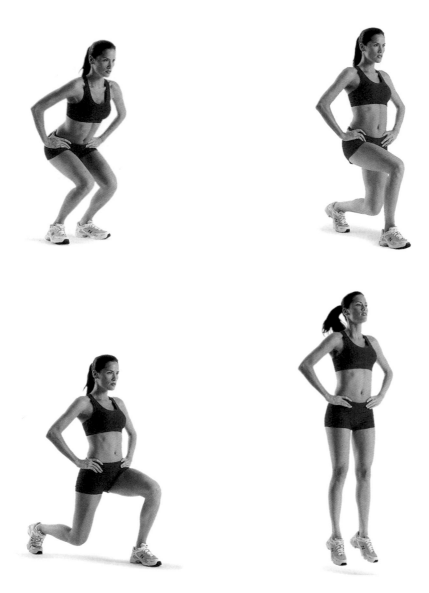

LEG CIRCUIT RACE

You race against the clock. Stand with your feet shoulder-width apart. Start by doing 20 body-weight squats, lowering your body until your thighs are parallel to the floor, at a rate of 1 squat per second. Next, perform 10 forward lunges with each leg, then 10 reverse lunges with each leg. (Again, aim for 1 repetition per second.) Finally, do 10 squat jumps—push off explosively so your feet leave the floor at the top of the move. Try to complete this routine in 75 seconds.

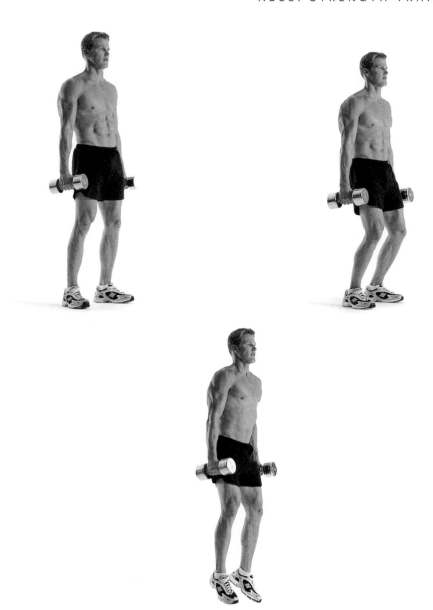

JUMP SQUAT

Use a pair of dumbbells that total about 30 percent of the weight you can squat one time. Hold the dumbbells at arm's length next to your thighs, your palms facing each other. Dip your knees slightly—as if you were about to leap—then explosively jump as high as you can. When you land, reset quickly and then jump again. Do 6 to 8 repetitions.

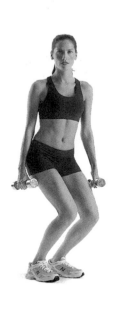

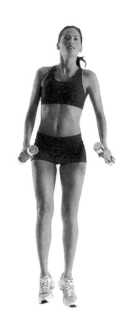

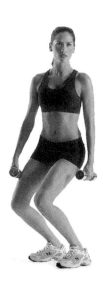

MOGUL TWIST SQUAT

Grab a pair of dumbbells and stand with your feet and lower body turned 45 degrees to your left, thighs halfway to horizontal. Jump and turn your lower body and upper body in opposite directions, landing with your lower body turned to the right.

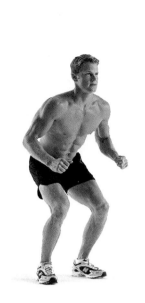
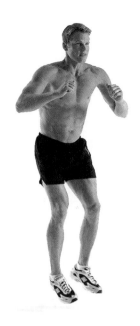
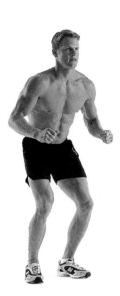

LINE JUMP

Stand next to a line (imaginary or real) with your feet next to each other and your knees slightly bent. Hop over the line with both feet. As soon as your feet touch the ground, hop back as fast as possible.

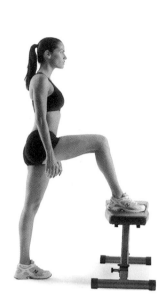
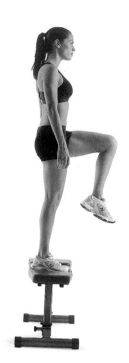

FRONT STEP-UP

Use a step (or bench) that's high enough so your thigh is parallel to the floor when your foot is on the step. Place your right foot on the step and push yourself up until your right leg is straight, then raise your left foot up. Step back down, left foot first, followed by your right.

VARIATION: *Stand sideways next to the step instead of facing it.*

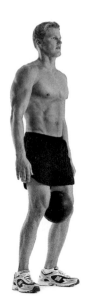
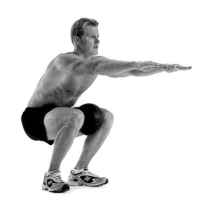

BALL SQUAT

Hold a medicine ball or a basketball between your knees as you perform the exercise. Keep your upper body as straight as possible and lower yourself until your thighs are parallel to the floor, then return to a standing position. TIP: You can either keep your hands on your sides or extend your arms forward for balance.

VARIATION: *Instead of using a ball, position a rubber belt, tube, or band just above your knees and spread your knees as you squat.*

"THANKS, ABS DIET!"

STEVE RAKOWSKI

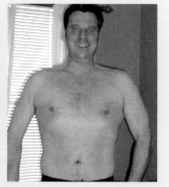

WEIGHT, WEEK 1: 225
WEIGHT, WEEK 6: 195

"I turned 40 in January, I quit smoking and drinking and started the program. I know I don't have the 6-pack abs yet, but this program changed my life. I am working out at the gym all the time and feeling great."

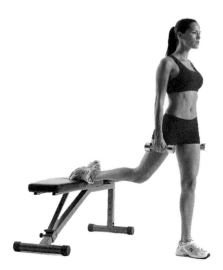
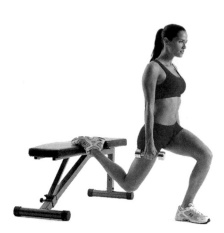

BULGARIAN SPLIT SQUAT

Hold a pair of dumbbells and stand about 3 feet in front of a bench. Place your right foot behind you on the bench so that only your instep is resting on it. Lower your body until your left knee is bent 90 degrees and your right knee nearly touches the floor. Your left lower leg should be perpendicular to the floor, and your torso should remain upright. Push yourself back to the starting position as quickly as you can. Finish 8 to 10 repetitions, then repeat the lift, this time with your left foot resting on the bench while your right leg does the work.

"THANKS, ABS DIET!"

DARREN DAURIO

WEIGHT, WEEK 1: 166
WEIGHT, WEEK 6: 153

"I always struggled to keep my waist size down. It seemed like the older I got, the more my waist size increased. After failing to achieve real results from expensive diets, I finally found a program that was reasonable, practical, enjoyable, and affordable. I finally have the abs I always wanted."

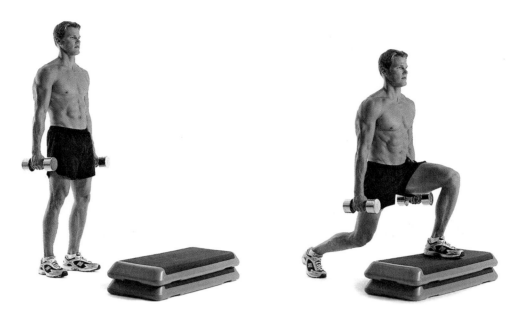

STEP LUNGE

Stand about 3 feet from an exercise step (or stair) with your feet about 6 inches apart. Hold two dumb-bells at your sides, your palms facing in. Keeping your back straight, step forward with your left foot and place it on the step. Lean forward until your left thigh is parallel to the floor. Then push yourself back to the starting position and repeat with your right leg.

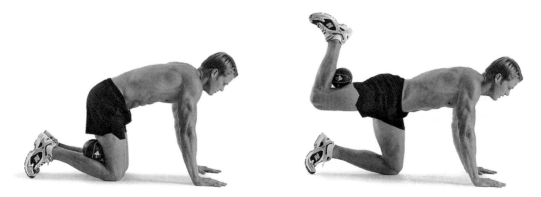

FIRE HYDRANT

Kneel on all fours on a mat and place a small medicine ball behind your right knee. Squeeze your leg muscles so that the ball stays locked in place. Keeping your back flat and your head down, slowly raise your right leg until the thigh is parallel to the floor. (The leg should form a right angle.) Pause, lower your leg to the starting position and repeat. Complete the set, then repeat with your left leg.

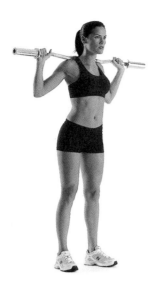 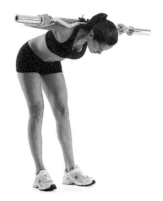

STIFF-LEG GOOD MORNING

Stand with a barbell on your shoulders, your feet shoulder-width apart, and your knees bent slightly. Maintain this knee angle throughout the move. Bend forward at the hips as far as you can without losing the flat or slightly arched posture in your lower back. Contract your glutes and push your hips forward to return to the starting position. Do 8 to 10 repetitions.

"THANKS, ABS DIET!"

DAVID GARTRELL

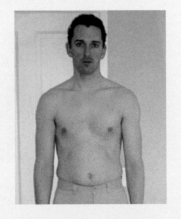 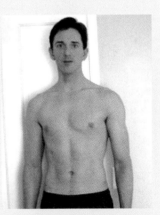

WEIGHT, WEEK 1: 186
WEIGHT, WEEK 6: 171

"My wife wasn't the only one who got bigger as we were expecting our first child. With all the planning and worrying (and ice cream cravings), diet and exercise took a back seat. But once our son arrived, I knew I needed to shape up, and the Abs Diet has been the perfect way to shed fat and gain some much-needed energy. I can see my abs for the first time, and I feel great!"

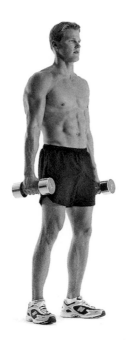
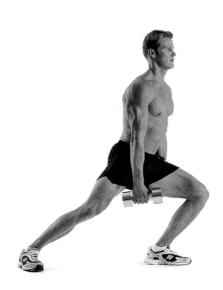

FRONT-ANGLE DUMBBELL LUNGE

Stand with your feet shoulder-width apart and hold a dumbbell in each hand, arms down at your sides. Step out with your left foot, placing it slightly forward and a few feet to the left. Lean onto your left leg and bend your left knee until your left thigh is almost parallel to the floor, then push back up to the starting position. Repeat the move, this time stepping out with your right foot. Do 8 to 10 repetitions on each leg.

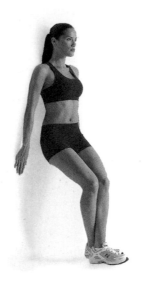 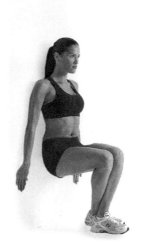

ONE-LEGGED WALL SQUAT

Stand with your back against a wall, your feet about 18 inches in front of you. Tuck your right foot behind your left calf, then perform a squat on one leg. Do 8 to 10 repetitions, then switch legs.

"THANKS, ABS DIET!"

ERIC BROOKS

WEIGHT, WEEK 1: 212
WEIGHT, WEEK 6: 195

"The Abs Diet has given me the opportunity to have the body of my youth. One that looks great, has the energy to play with my 7 children, and has the confidence to turn up the heat with my beautiful wife. Unlike other diets, the Abs Diet has taught me how to eat. 'Show a man what to eat, and he'll be fit for a day. Teach him *why* to eat, and he'll be fit for life.'"

CHEST

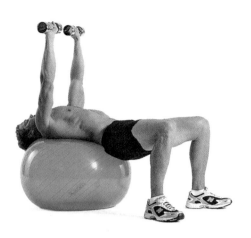
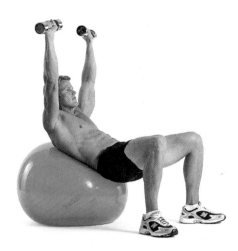

SWISS BALL PRESS WITH CRUNCH

Lie with your back, shoulders, and head in contact with a Swiss ball and hold a pair of dumbbells (elbows bent) above your shoulders. Press the weights up until your arms are straight. Then do a crunch by lifting your shoulder blades off the ball. Pause, lower your shoulders, then lower the weights. Do 8 to 10 repetitions.

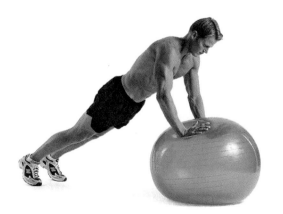
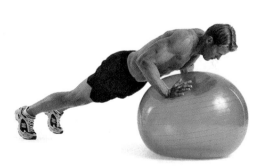

SWISS BALL INCLINE/DECLINE PUSHUP

With your toes on the floor, assume the standard pushup position, but place your hands on a Swiss ball directly under your shoulders. Bend your arms until your chest touches the ball. Pause, then push yourself back up to the starting position. Do 8 to 12 repetitions.

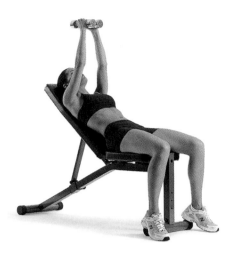
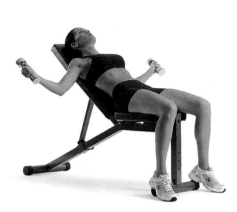

CHEST FLY

Lie on your back on an incline bench with a dumbbell in each hand. With your arms bent slightly, raise your arms straight above your chest, palms facing each other. Slowly lower the dumbbells in an arc down and away from your body. Pause, then slowly raise the weights, following the same curving path, until the weights are again above your chest. Do 8 to 10 repetitions.

"THANKS, ABS DIET!"

JONATHAN ROMAN

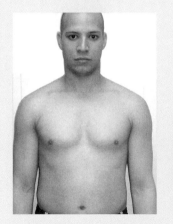
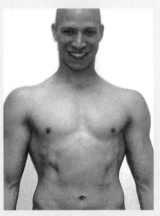

WEIGHT, WEEK 1: 192
WEIGHT, WEEK 6: 173

"The Abs Diet brought to me perseverance, discipline, and a change of character that will stay with me the rest of my life. Now I'm focused and determined, and confidence has led to an attitude that I can overcome any obstacle in my path. An attitude of purpose also revealed to me a new aspect on life, increasing my self-esteem and knowing that anything I put my will into is not impossible for me to accomplish."

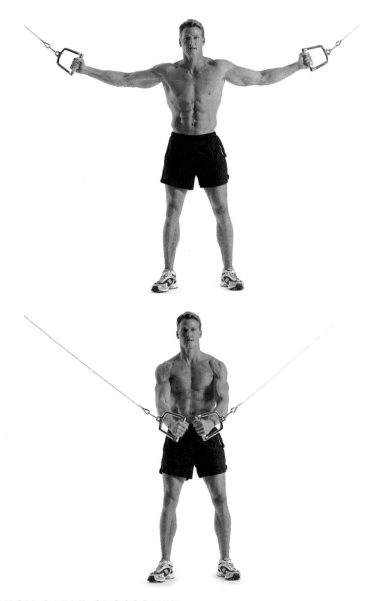

STANDING HIGH-CABLE CROSSOVER

Attach two stirrup handles to the high cable-crossover station and stand sideways to the weight stack. Grab the left handle with your left hand and the right handle with your right hand, and stand in the middle of the station. You may also want to step back; it's best to start with tension in the cables so there's resistance throughout the movement. Pull your shoulder blades back and keep your elbows slightly bent. Pull the handles down in a wide arc in front of your body until your hands touch each other in front of your midsection. Pause, then return to the starting position. Do 8 to 12 repetitions.

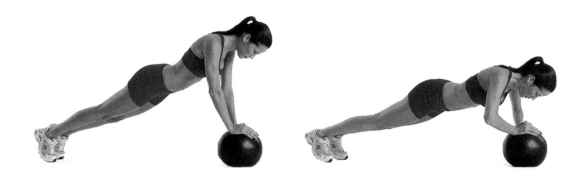

MEDICINE BALL PUSHUP

Kneel and place your hands along the sides of a medicine ball, spreading your fingers wide to help grip the surface (a soccer ball or basketball will also work). The space between your thumbs and index fingers should be diamond-shaped. Balance your weight on the ball, then slowly extend your legs behind you to assume the pushup position. Lower your body until your chest touches the ball. Pause, then slowly press yourself back up to the starting position. Do 8 to 10 repetitions.

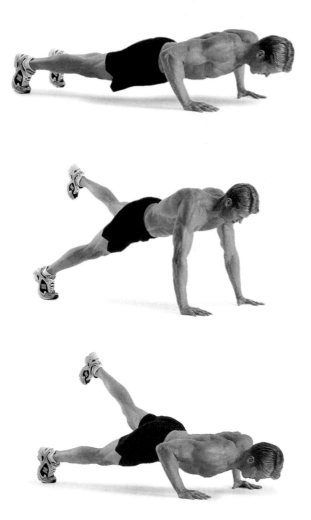

LEG-LIFT PUSHUP

Get into the down position of a pushup, your hands in line with your shoulders, about 6 inches away from your body. Set your feet hip-width apart. Push up by straightening your arms and raise your left leg as high as you can. Keep your leg raised while you perform a normal pushup by lowering your chest to the floor. Keep your back flat and your body rigid. Switch legs on each repetition. Do 8 to 10 repetitions.

SHOULDERS

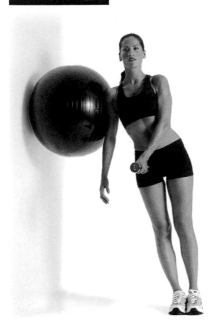 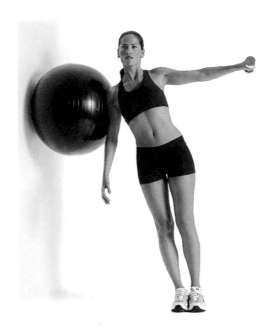

SWISS BALL LATERAL RAISES

Lean your right shoulder against a Swiss ball that's placed against a wall. Keeping your body straight, place your feet less than shoulder-width apart and far enough from the wall so that your body is at an angle from the floor. Hold a dumbbell in your left hand and let the hand hang across your body toward your right leg, palm facing the wall. Lift your arm up and out to your left until it forms a straight line with your shoulders. Pause, then slowly lower the weight back down. Do 12 repetitions with each arm.

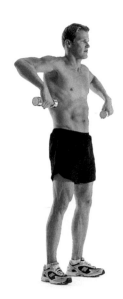
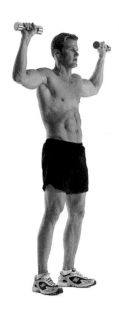

STANDING SCARECROW

Stand holding a light dumbbell (5 to 10 pounds) in each hand with your palms facing back and raise your upper arms so they're parallel to the floor with your elbows bent 90 degrees. (The weights should point down to the floor.) Keeping your elbows, wrists and upper arms locked, rotate the weights up over your head and as far back as you can. Pause, then slowly return to the starting position by rotating the weight down; keep your upper arms parallel to the floor. Do 8 repetitions.

"THANKS, ABS DIET!"

NICK RENDON

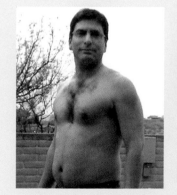
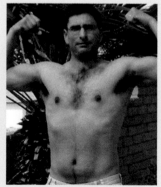

WEIGHT, WEEK 1: 192
WEIGHT, WEEK 6: 180

"All my pants fit loosely now. Heck, I had my wife buy me a pair of 33-inch pants and I could fit in 32s! I don't have the 6-pack yet, but I *will*. It has been a great life change without a huge change in my daily lifestyle."

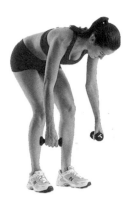
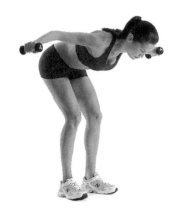

REAR LATERAL RAISE

Grab a pair of dumbbells and stand with your feet shoulder-width apart. Keeping your back flat, bend at your waist and knees until your upper body is almost parallel to the floor. Let the dumbbells hang at arm's length (elbows slightly bent), with your thumbs turned toward each other. Slowly raise the dumbbells as high as you can without changing the angle of your elbows. Pause, then lower the weights to the starting position, maintaining the elbow angle. Do 12 repetitions.

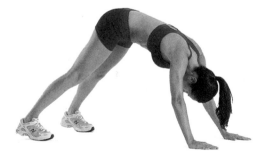
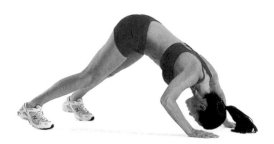

PIKE PUSHUPS

Start with your hands and feet flat on the floor (or your feet on a bench) and your butt as high as possible. Slowly lower your shoulders toward the floor until your head touches. Push back to the starting position. Do 8 to 10 repetitions.

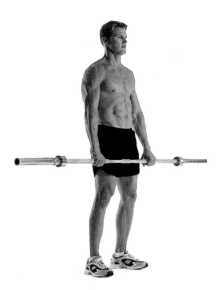
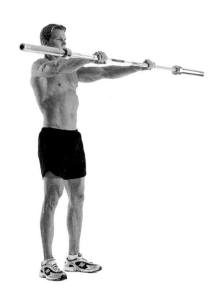

BARBELL FRONT RAISE

Stand with your feet shoulder-width apart and hold a barbell in front of your thighs. Your hands should be about shoulder-width apart, palms down. Keeping your back and arms straight, slowly raise the bar in an arc in front of your chest until your arms are parallel to the floor. Pause, then slowly lower the bar until your hands almost touch your thighs. Do 8 to 10 repetitions.

"THANKS, ABS DIET!"

MICHAEL WILFING

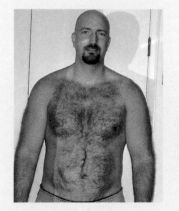
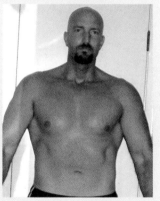

WEIGHT, WEEK 1: 260
WEIGHT, WEEK 6: 238

"I have been working out and dieting for years, but never achieved the results I have been striving for. But with the Abs Diet, I can truly say I have achieved those desired results. My waist is slimmer and tighter, and my overall muscularity is solid and tight. I have more energy and I look forward to each workout to strive for even better results. Thank you for the new me."

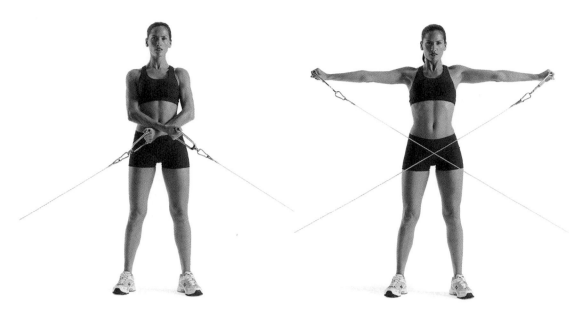

CABLE TWO-ARM RAISE

Stand between the weight of a cable-crossover station tower and use your right hand to grab the bottom handle that's to your left. Grab the opposite bottom handle with your left hand and stand with your arms down in front of you, the handles crossing below your waist. Keeping your arms straight but your elbows unlocked, slowly raise your arms out to the sides until they're parallel to the floor and your palms face down. Your body forms a T shape. Pause for 1 second, then slowly lower your arms to the starting position. Do 8 to 10 repetitions.

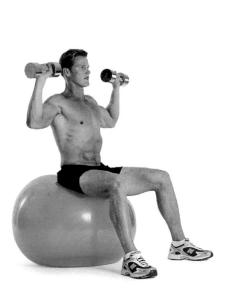
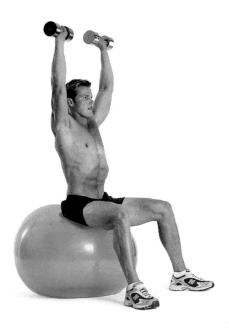

SWISS BALL PRESS

Sit on a Swiss ball with your feet flat on the floor. Grab dumbbells or a light barbell and hold the weight in front of your chest, hands spaced slightly more than shoulder-width apart. Slowly press the weights over your head until your arms are straight. Do 8 to 10 repetitions.

"THANKS, ABS DIET!"

TRAVIS HENCKEL

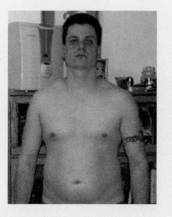
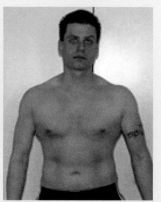

WEIGHT, WEEK 1: 185
WEIGHT, WEEK 6: 170

"The biggest change to my life has been the energy it has given me, allowing me to be more interactive with my family. I used to be sedentary. Now I actively play with my children and strive to keep everyone happy. My whole family has seen the positive changes in me, and all of us now exercise and stay active!"

BACK

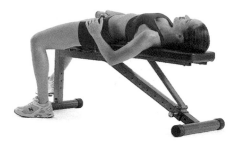 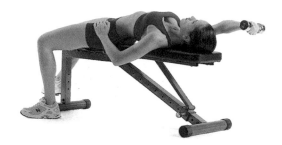

STRAIGHT-ARM ALTERNATING PULLOVER

Lie faceup on a bench with your right leg straight, the thigh flat on the bench. Keep your left foot on the floor. Hold a dumbbell in your right hand above your thigh, palm facing in. Keeping your arm straight, lift it up and back so it makes a 180-degree arc. Pause, then return to the starting position. Switch legs and hands after each set. Do 12 repetitions with each arm.

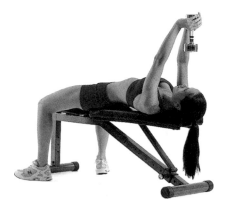 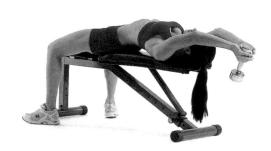

DUMBBELL PULLOVER

Grab a light dumbbell and lie flat on a bench. Wrapping your thumbs and forefingers in a diamond shape around the handle, use both hands to hold the weight vertically over your head. Keeping your elbows slightly bent, slowly lower the weight backward in an arc over your head until you feel a slight stretch in your sides and your upper arms are in line with your head. Pause, then slowly pull the weight back over your chest. Do 8 to 10 repetitions.

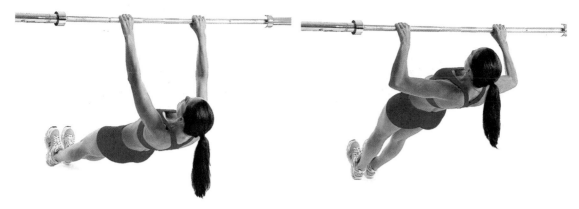

REVERSE PUSHUP

Secure a bar 3 or 4 feet above the floor on a Smith machine. Lie under the bar and grab it with a shoulder-width, overhand grip. Hang at arm's length from the bar with your body straight and your heels on the floor or a stability ball. Keep your body rigid and pull your chest to the bar. Pause, then lower yourself back to the starting position. Do 8 to 10 repetitions.

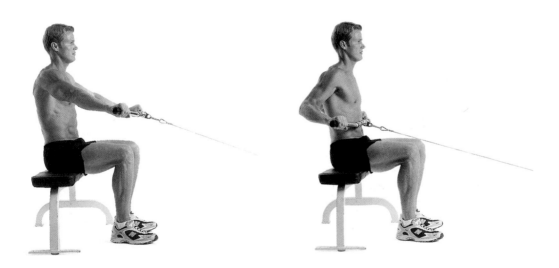

WIDE-GRIP SEATED ROW

Attach a long straight bar to a low-cable rowing station. Sit on the bench and grab the bar with an overhand grip, your hands slightly more than shoulder-width apart. Slowly pull the bar to your midsection. Slowly let the bar pull your arms out in front of you. Do 8 to 10 repetitions.

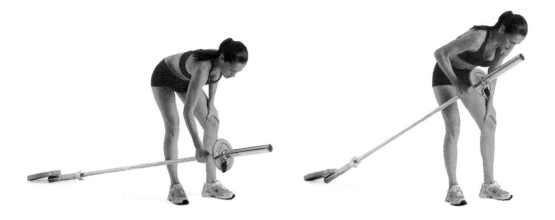

ONE-HAND BENT-OVER ROW BAR

Place a bar on the floor with one end resting in a corner. Attach a few light weights to the other end. With your back facing the corner, stand to the left of the bar and bend forward so that your torso is almost parallel to the floor. Grab the barbell directly behind the weight with your right hand. Your left hand can rest on your left knee for stability. Slowly pull the bar up toward your right side until the weights touch your chest. Lower the bar to within an inch or two of the floor. Do 10 to 12 repetitions with each arm.

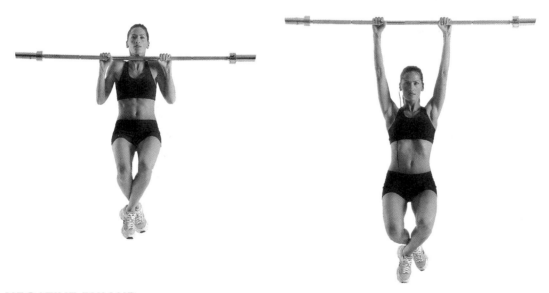

NEGATIVE PULLUP

Using a step (or a boost from a partner), hoist your chest to a pullup bar. Then lower yourself slowly—try for a count of 12 before your arms are straight. Complete a set of 6 to 8 repetitions.

BICEPS

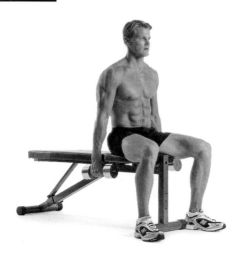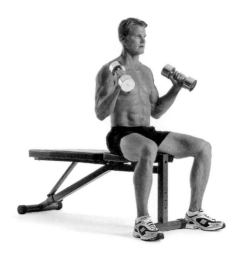

HAMMER CURLS

Sit on the end of a bench with a dumbbell in each hand. Let your arms hang straight down, palms facing each other. Slowly curl both weights up towards your shoulders. Bring the weights to your shoulders and squeeze your biceps. Slowly lower the weights until your arms are straight again. Do 8 to 10 repetitions.

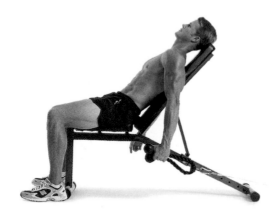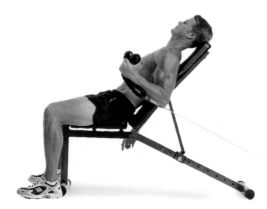

LOW-CABLE HAMMER CURL

Place an incline bench at a 45-degree angle in front of a low-cable station and turn it so your back faces the weight station. Attach a rope handle to the low pulley, sit down, and grab both ends with one hand. Your arm should hang straight down from your body. Without moving your upper arm, bend your elbow and curl the rope toward your chest. Pause, then bring your arm back into the starting position. Afterward, switch arms. Do 8 to 10 repetitions with each arm.

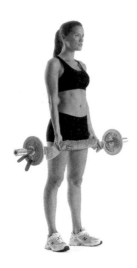
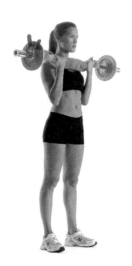

FAT-GRIP BARBELL CURL

Wrap two hand towels around a barbell and grab the towel-wrapped bar with an underhand, shoulder-width grip. Hold the bar at arm's length in front of your thighs. Without moving your upper arms forward or changing your posture, slowly curl the bar as high as you can. Then, without pausing, take 3 seconds to lower it back to the starting position. Do 8 to 10 repetitions.

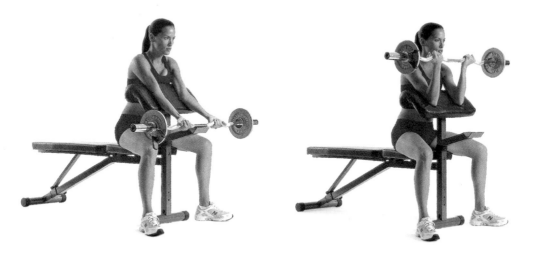

PREACHER CURL

Sit at a preacher-curl station and grab a pair of light dumbbells or an EZ-curl bar with an underhand grip. Rest your upper arms on the slanted pad in front of you. Keeping your back straight, slowly curl the bar up until your forearms are just short of perpendicular to the floor. Then lower the weight back down. Do 8 to 10 repetitions.

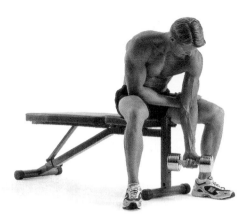 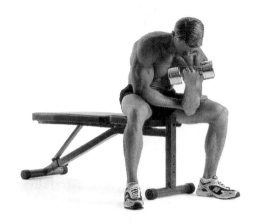

CONCENTRATION CURL

Sit on the edge of a bench with a dumbbell in your left hand, your legs spread out to the sides. Rest the back of your left arm against the inside of your left thigh. Hold the weight with an underhand grip and let it hang straight down. Rest your right hand on your left thigh. Curl the weight up toward your left shoulder. Pause, then lower the weight to the starting position. Do 8 to 10 repetitions with each arm.

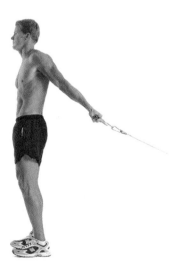 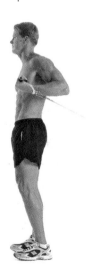

BEHIND-THE-BACK ONE-ARM CABLE CURL

Stand with your back to the weight stack of a cable station and grab the bottom stirrup handle with one hand. Take a few steps away from the stack so there is resistance and your arm is roughly 45 degrees from horizontal. Slowly curl the handle forward and up until your hand reaches the side of your chest. Then lower your arm to the starting position. This stretches your biceps beyond the usual range of motion. Do 8 to 10 repetitions with each arm.

TRICEPS

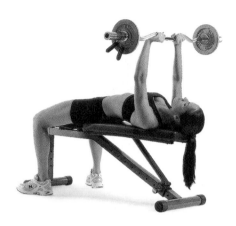 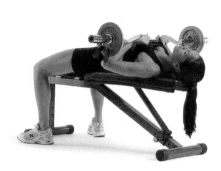

EZ-CURL BAR BENCH PRESS

Lie on your back on a bench and grab an EZ-curl barbell with an overhand grip, your hands less than shoulder-width apart and arms extended. Slowly lower the bar to your chest. Pause, then press the weight back overhead; keep your elbows flexed. Do 10 to 12 repetitions.

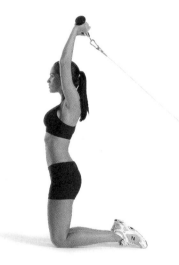 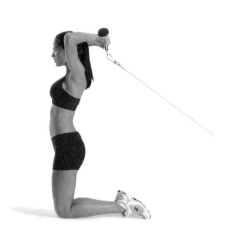

KNEELING CABLE EXTENSION

Attach a V-bar to a low-pulley cable and kneel with your back to the stack. Turn around to grab both handles, then face forward and straighten your arms overhead. (The bottom of the V should be pointing down.) Keeping your upper arms stationary, slowly bend your elbows and lower your hands behind your neck. Reverse the motion, straightening your arms and locking your elbows at the top to contract the triceps. Do 10 to 12 repetitions.

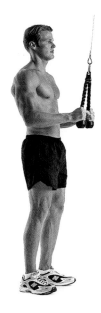
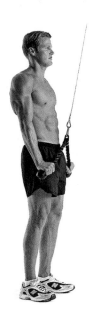

ROPE PULLDOWN

Use a rope attachment instead of a bar on a high-pulley. Facing the pulley, grab each end of the rope so your palms face each other. Pull the rope down until your arms are straight, turning your wrists outward at the bottom. Do 10 to 12 repetitions.

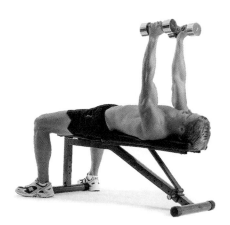
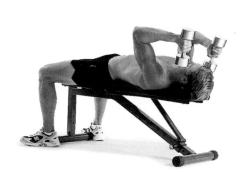

LYING DUMBBELL EXTENSION

Lying on your back on a bench, hold a set of dumbbells overhead with your arms straight and your palms facing each other. Keeping your upper arms stationary, slowly lower the weights toward your shoulders until they reach the sides of your head. Pause, then slowly press the weights back up, but keep your elbows unlocked. Do 10 to 12 repetitions.

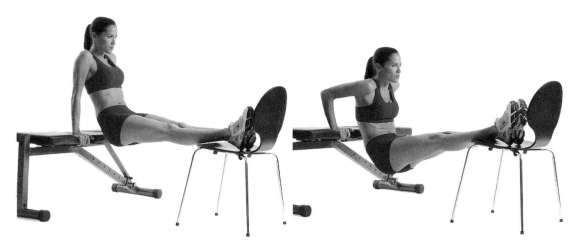

BENCH DIP

Stand with your back to a bench and place your hands on the edge, fingers pointing toward your lower back. Place your feet on a chair or another bench a few feet in front of you. Keeping your hands in place, slowly step forward until your legs are extended in front of you, knees slightly bent. Your arms should be straight, elbows unlocked, supporting your weight. Slowly bend your arms to lower yourself as far as you can and bring your butt as close to the floor as possible. Press yourself back up to the starting position. Do 10 to 12 repetitions.

ABS FACT

15

Number of beats higher that circuit training raises your heart rate, compared to running at 60 to 70 percent of your maximum heart rate

ABS DIET SUCCESS STORY

"IT'S EASY—EVEN IF YOU TRAVEL"

Name: John Messamore

Age: 29

Height: 5'10"

Starting weight: 216

Six weeks later: 187

Starting waist size: 37"

Waist size six weeks later: 31"

When John Messamore took his "before" pictures, he didn't realize he had that much around the middle.

"Looking at my pictures was a real eye opener," he says. "I always dressed well and people just thought I was a big guy."

Messamore actually started the diet while he was on the road for business—meaning that he had to eat out for every meal. Ordering grilled fish, eggs, some protein shakes, and fruit, he was still able to see results.

"With the 12 Powerfoods, it's pretty easy to incorporate into your life, especially if you travel a lot," says Messamore, who traveled 2 out of the first 6 weeks he was on the plan.

"I think the cheat day helped. It gave me something to look forward to," he says. "As I progressed more and more, it wasn't that I wanted the cheat so much. The cheat day is a goal: I just have to make it until Saturday."

Messamore also stuck to the Abs Diet circuit—with special attention to his often-neglected legs—and found it a challenging way to build muscle and get his heart rate up. Toward the end of the 6 weeks, he kicked the cardio up a bit and really targeted his abs—and, even though he had always worked out, he ended up swimming in his clothes.

"The diet is unbelievable," he says. "I gained more energy, focus, muscle, strength, confidence, professional success, and drive—especially in the bedroom."

Chapter 4

ABS3: SPEED INTERVALS

Get Your Heart Rate Up to Get Your Waist Size Down

SLOWING WAY DOWN AND SPEEDING WAY UP AGAIN may get you in trouble on the interstate (and in the bedroom), but when it comes to cardiovascular exercise, it's the key for weight loss. I've already explained that speed interval workouts—workouts that alternate high-intensity levels with lower-intensity effort—help your body burn calories long after you've stopped working out. You can use interval workouts any way you want—running, cycling, swimming, on elliptical trainers, even walking if you alternate a speed walk and slow walk. To keep your workouts fresh and to keep your body guessing, you can also vary the intensity levels in different combinations. (If you use exercise machines, don't choose the interval workout; choose the manual one and create your own intensities by adjusting it yourself. It'll give you greater control over the speeds and will help you burn fat faster.)

The best part? You'll derive benefits in as little as a 20-minute interval workout. As you build up endurance and strength, you can add time to your workout, and you can add an extra interval workout per week. But don't do it more than twice a week. You may burn calories, but you'll also burn out.

I'm presenting many options here based on various machines and approaches, but just like in strength-training workouts, you can tailor the principles to concoct your own interval workout. So, for example, the workout on the treadmill may work just as well on a stairclimber. The following programs are preset plans, but they should also give you ideas for ways to build your own high-intensity interval training sessions.

ABS FACT

47

Percentage by which you decrease the risk of dementia by doing 3 hours of walking a week

The Great Pyramids Interval

This pyramid structure allows you to start with short bursts of speed, and then you'll peak at the longest surge of energy in the middle of your workout before coming back down.

3 to 5 minutes warmup

30 seconds high intensity

1 minute low intensity

45 seconds high intensity

1 minute low intensity

1 minute high intensity

1 minute low intensity

90 seconds high intensity

1 minute low intensity

1 minute high intensity

1 minute low intensity

45 seconds high intensity

1 minute low intensity

30 seconds high intensity

3 to 5 minutes cooldown

The Minute-Man Interval

The following is a typical interval workout you can use with any cardiovascular exercise. You alternate one period of low intensity with the same period of higher intensity.

> 3 to 5 minutes warmup (light jog, low intensity, gradually increasing at the end of the warmup period)
>
> 1 minute moderate or high intensity followed by 1 minute low intensity (repeat 6 to 8 times)
>
> 3 to 5 minutes cooldown (light jog, low intensity, gradually decreasing by the end of the cooldown period)

The All-Star Interval

Sports are as unpredictable as Jon Stewart's mouth. This interval simulates some of that unpredictability by having you doing different times and different intensities. You can

CLASSES IN SESSION

If you prefer taking group classes, these are three worth trying.

In some exercise classes, the only workout you get is for your eyes. But in these sessions, you can work your heart and your muscles—to get an all-around effective interval workout.

Sports Conditioning/Boot Camp: Constant action of intervals, plyometric exercises, and speed drills.

Cool move to steal: Hand stepping. Get into pushup position—your hands slightly wider than and in line with your shoulders—in front of a 3- to 6-inch-high step or at the base of your stairs. With your arms straight (but not locked) and your back flat, place your left hand on the step, followed by your right. Then immediately reverse the movement, placing your left hand back on the floor first. That's 1 repetition. Do 3 sets of 12 repetitions between sets of 12 regular pushups.

Kickboxing: Series of punches, kicks, and plyometric moves that mimic real boxing.

Cool move to steal: High knee jump. In one move, jump as high as you can and bring your knees as close to your chest as possible. Do 10 repetitions at the end of your leg workout, or superset them with squats, performing the two exercises back-to-back with no rest between sets.

Spinning: Stationary cycling at different speeds and levels of resistance.

Cool move to steal: The uphill interval. Start with an easy tension on the bike—about 40 percent of your maximum effort—while you maintain a cadence of 80 to 120 revolutions per minute. Increase the tension one notch every 30 seconds until it's similar to the amount of resistance you'd feel if you were cycling up a very steep hill. Then work your way back down the pyramid by reducing the resistance by one notch every 30 seconds.

mix and match the orders and repetitions as much as you want. Rest longer after the periods in which you use the most energy.

3 to 5 minutes warmup

2 minutes moderate or high intensity followed by 2 minutes low intensity (repeat once)

30 seconds high intensity followed by 30 seconds low intensity (repeat 4 times)

60-yard sprints (or 10 seconds if not running) followed by 90 seconds rest (repeat 6 to 10 times)

3 to 5 minutes cooldown

The Knee-Saving Interval

Elliptical machines are like security guards at a reggae concert—they're easy on your joints. Researchers at the University of Mississippi found that elliptical trainers provide the same cardiovascular benefits as treadmill running, without the impact on your ankles, knees, and hips. Instead of holding on to the handles, pump your arms (as if you were running). For this interval, alternate intervals of high resistance with those of high speed.

3 to 5 minutes warmup

2 minutes high resistance, lower stride pace

2 minutes low resistance, high stride pace

Repeat 5 times

3 to 5 minutes cooldown

The Go-Row Interval

Unlike most other cardiovascular machines, rowing machines are the massage therapists of cardio workouts—they work both your upper and lower body. One trick: On the back stroke, your knees should be almost completely straight before you squeeze your shoulder blades together and pull the handle to your sternum. Your back should stay in its naturally arched position during the entire movement. For this interval, set the machine at moderate resistance.

3 to 5 minutes warmup

10 power strokes: pulling the handle as hard and fast as you can

1 minute easy rowing

15 power strokes

1 minute easy rowing

20 power strokes

1 minute easy rowing

Repeat circuit 4 to 5 times

3 to 5 minutes cooldown

The Climb Every Machine Interval

Stepping can be a great way to work your heart and add lean muscle to your legs. If you're doing it on a machine, don't lean on the handles—you'll burn 20 percent fewer calo-

WHAT IS "METABOLISM" ANYWAY?

A lot of people throw around the word "metabolism" the way the Sopranos throw around F-words. Metabolism is the rate at which your body burns its way through calories simply to keep itself alive—to keep your organs and systems functioning. Your body is actually burning calories all the time, even when the only muscles you're moving are in your thumbs. The average woman burns about 10 calories per pound of body weight ever day; the average man, 11 calories per pound. These are the three ways in which your body burns calories:

• **The thermic effect of eating.** Between 10 and 30 percent of the calories you expend each day are burned by the simple act of digesting your food. Your body uses more calories to digest protein (about 25 calories burned for every 100 calories consumed) than it does to digest fats and carbohydrates (10 to 15 calories burned for every 100 calories consumed).

• **Exercise and movement.** Another 10 to 15 percent of your calorie burn comes from moving your muscles, whether you're pressing weights overhead, running to catch the bus, or flicking between commercials.

• **Basal metabolism.** Your basal, or resting, metabolism refers to the calories you're burning when you're doing nothing at all. In fact, between 60 and 80 percent of your daily calories are burned up just doing nothing. That's because even at rest, your body is constantly in motion: Your heart is beating, your lungs are breathing, and your cells are dividing all the time.

ries. Pump your arms instead. Or turn around. A study in the *Archives of Physical Medicine and Rehabilitation* found that facing away from the console burned more calories than the traditional method. Try this escalating interval:

3 to 5 minutes warmup

Increase resistance by one level every 2 minutes

Increase 6 to 8 times

3 to 5 minutes cooldown

The Pedal-Pushing Interval

A lot of times, stationary bikes are the couches of the gym—you see a lot of people not working very hard on them. You can avoid being lulled into a dull workout by using this interval. One tip: Many cyclists develop lower-back pain because of their posture. Stand up every few minutes and pedal as if you were climbing a hill for 60 seconds. It'll take the pressure off your lower back and force you to use different muscles. A good speed workout:

3 to 5 minutes warmup

90 seconds pedaling at 95-percent maximum effort

90 seconds at 40 percent of full effort

1 minute pedaling at 95-percent maximum effort

1 minute at 40 percent of full effort

30 seconds pedaling at 95-percent maximum effort

30 seconds at 40 percent of full effort

4 minutes at 60 percent of full effort

Repeat set of intervals once

3 to 5 minutes cooldown

The Do-Run-Run Interval

Score one for the treadmill: A study in *Medicine and Science in Sports and Exercise* determined that the treadmill burns calories

ABS FACT

10

Number of yards farther golfers who did medicine ball exercises drove the ball, compared to those who did light machine workouts at the highest rate of any exercise machine. (If you want to mimic road running, raise the incline of the treadmill to 1 percent before starting your run. Researchers in England found that it's the degree of treadmill elevation that most closely approximates outdoor running.) You can do lots of different interval options on it—alternating between running and walking, between faster and slower, between higher and lower inclines. Here's one suggestion for an ascending and descending program:

3 to 5 minutes warmup

2 minutes, speed that's 2 minutes per mile slower than average pace, 1 percent incline

2 minutes, same speed, 4 percent incline

2 minutes, same speed, 6 percent incline

2 minutes, same speed, 8 percent incline

2 minutes, same speed, 10 percent incline

TREAD CAREFULLY

Running on a mechanical belt is a wee bit different than running on solid asphalt. If you want the closet simulation to outdoor running, set the treadmill at a 1-percent incline. Upgrade the incline to set an even faster perceived pace.

TREADMILL MILE PACE		HOW THE EFFORT FEELS		
	FLAT	1 PERCENT	2 PERCENT	3 PERCENT
5:00	5:21	5:06	4:53	4:41
6:00	6:26	6:08	5:52	5:37
7:00	7:30	7:09	6:50	6:33
8:00	8:34	8:11	7:49	7:29
9:00	9:39	9:12	8:48	8:25
10:00	10:43	10:13	9:46	9:22
11:00	11:47	11:15	10:45	10:18
12:00	12:52	12:16	11:44	11:14

2 minutes, same speed, 8 percent incline

2 minutes, same speed, 6 percent incline

2 minutes, same speed, 4 percent incline

2 minutes, same speed, 2 percent incline

3 to 5 minutes cooldown

The Fan in the Stands Intervals

High school did a lot for your heart. (Remember the Homecoming queen?) Now, it can do even more. Find yourself a football stadium that's open to the public and turn your interval circuit into a strength-and-speed workout that will burn fat as well as strengthen your legs and your upper body.

Circuit 1

Run to the top row of the stands, touching every step; jog down; immediately do 20 pushups. Repeat the stair climbs three more times, doing a different one of these exercises after each: 20 squats, 20 incline or decline pushups (put your hands on either a higher or lower step than your feet), 20 crunches. Then rest 2 minutes.

Circuit 2

Sprint up the stairs, touching every step and exploding off each stride. Jog down and do 10 squat jumps (jump straight from a squat). Repeat three more times doing one of these after each: 20 wide-grip pushups, 20 walking lunges, 10 squat jumps. Rest 2 minutes.

Circuit 3

Climb the stairs three at a time, as a series of step-ups. Put your leading leg on the higher step, then bring your trailing leg up alongside it; lead with the other leg for the next step. Jog back down and do 30 crunches. Repeat three more times, with one of these after each: 20 lower-back supermans (on your belly, lift your outstretched arms and legs), 30 crunches, and 20 more supermans.

STRETCHING: THE TRUTH

These moves will make you more flexible.

Seems like stretching is the gun-control issue of the exercise world. Some are in favor; others are adamantly opposed. But here's what you need to know: Stretching is not the same as warming up. Warming up needs to be dynamic—that is, you need to get your muscles moving in the form of walking, cycling, jumping jacks, or lunges. That will help prevent injuries by slowly increasing blood flow to your muscles so they can prepare for the exercise. The stretching that you're used to seeing (bend down and touch toes) is more static, in that your muscles move into one position and stay there. To prevent injury and help increase your flexibility (both are good things), that's best done after your muscles are warm—at the *end* of a warmup or after a workout. You already know about the classic stretches—touch toes to stretch hamstrings, butterfly to stretch your groin and inner thighs. But here are some that are both a little static and little dynamic, which will help you warm up as well as increase and maintain your muscular flexibility.

For hamstrings, calves, lower back, and glutes: Bend forward from the waist, with your legs straight and your hands on the floor. (You'll probably need to begin with your hands a couple of feet in front of you in a wider V-shape.) Keeping your legs straight, walk your hands forward as far as possible. Hold for 3 to 5 seconds. Then take tiny steps to walk your feet up to your hands. Hold again for 3 to 5 seconds. Repeat for a set of 5.

For hip flexors, quadriceps, and abs: Lie on your stomach with your arms straight out at your sides and your legs straight, so your body forms a T. Keeping your arms still, thrust your left heel toward your right hand by squeezing your glutes (your butt) and bending your knee. Bring your leg back to the starting position, then try to touch your right heel to your left hand. Do 5 reps with each leg.

For back, shoulders, and triceps: Lie facedown on a Swiss ball with your abs drawn in and your arms hanging down, holding light dumbbells. Raise your arms straight back until they're in line with your body and pull your shoulder blades down and together. Hold the stretch for 2 to 3 seconds, then return to the starting position and repeat 10 times.

The Hard-Hitting Interval

If you have a heavy bag in your gym or basement, you can do a rare interval workout—one that emphasizes, tones, and strengthens your upper body. You'll need hand wraps and gloves—and a timer or a clock with a second hand, since it'll be hard to use a sports watch with gloves on. Pound away, and watch the pounds go away.

Starting position: Stand about 2½ feet away from the bag with your feet shoulder-width apart, left foot toward the bag at 12 o'clock, right foot at 2–3 o'clock (for righties; reverse for lefties). Keep right on the balls of your feet and bob around the bag to keep moving. Aim to throw 70 to 80 punches per round.

3 to 5 minutes warmup

2 to 3 minutes straight left jabs

1 minute rest

2 to 3 minutes right crosses

1 minute rest

2 to 3 minutes straight left jabs and right crosses (three to five jabs for every cross)

1 minute rest

2 to 3 minutes right and left hooks

1 minute rest

2 to 3 minutes all punches

3 to 5 minutes cooldown

How to Throw Punches

All directions are for righties from the starting position; switch directions for lefties. With all punches, visualize punching through the bag to follow through.

Left Jab: With your left hand at your chin, extend and snap your whole left arm toward the bag, stepping to it with your left foot.

Right Cross: With your left hand at your chin and your right hand to the side of your face, pivot your upper body and punch with your right arm across your body to stroke the bag.

Hooks: Bend forward and drop your arms to chest level. Pivot away from the bag, then as you punch by hooking your arm, pivot back toward the bag.

The Fast-Track Interval

Tired of the stadium stairs? Then hit the track; the quarter-mile loop offers the perfect setup for running intervals—not only because of the distance, but also because most tracks have softer, more cushioning surfaces than blacktop or concrete. You have lots of options, but here are three.

Repeats

3 to 5 minutes warmup

Run twice around track (800 meters) at a pace 10 seconds faster than mile pace

Jog 1 lap

Repeat sequence 3 times

3 to 5 minutes cooldown

THE WATER RULES

You know that water is good for more than plants and spring break T-shirts. It's also imperative you get some during your workout. Here's how to make sure you're well-watered.

Drinking	Start drinking water at least 15 minutes before starting. Drink 8 ounces for every 20 minutes of exercise.
Sweat Rate	Weigh yourself before and after a workout and subtract the weight of any water you drank while exercising. If the before-and-after difference is . . .
	• 2 percent of your body weight, your athletic performance suffered
	• 3 to 4 percent of your body weight, there are potential health risks, including elevated heart rate and body temperature
Refueling	For every pound of body weight you've lost during your workout, drink 16 ounces of water. Then remember that guideline for your next workout. So if you're 2 pounds lighter after an hour-long run, drink 32 ounces more before or during your next run.
The Toilet Test	If your urine looks more like iced tea than lemonade, you're de-hydrated. The closer to clear, the better.

In-and-outs

3 to 5 minutes warmup

200 meters (½ lap) at fastest mile pace

200 meters jog

Repeat for 2 miles

3 to 5 minutes cooldown

Advanced: On the football field inside the track

Warmup (10-minute jog/stretch)

Ten 100s (100-yard sprints in 15 to 18 seconds, interspersed with 30-to-35-second rests)

Eight 80s (80-yard sprints in 11 to 15 seconds, with 20-to-25-second rests)

Six 60s (60-yard sprints in 8 to 11 seconds, with 15-to-20-second rests)

Four 40s (40-yard sprints in 5 to 8 seconds, with 10-to-15-second rests)

Cooldown (10-minute jog/stretch)

The Please the Court Interval

Sure, practicing free throws and pretending to be Artis Gilmore may be fun and all when you're by yourself, but you can also use the court to get an interval workout that's made many a baller get into game shape.

3 to 5 minutes warmup

Fours: Run four lengths of a basketball court as hard as you can, with the goal of finishing in under 24 seconds. Rest 40 seconds and repeat 8 to 12 times. Then rest 2 minutes.

17s: Run sideline to sideline 17 times. The challenge is changing direction. Try to finish in about a minute. Rest 2 minutes; repeat for a total of two or three runs.

Suicides: Starting at one baseline of a basketball court, run to the near free-throw line and back, then continue back and forth to the mid-court line, the opposite free-throw line, and the opposite baseline. Try to run the whole thing in 30 to 33 seconds, then rest for a minute. Complete three to six suicides.

3 to 5 minutes cooldown

The Fancy-Footwork Interval

You don't have to be a salsa dancer to benefit from great footwork. Agility drills not only raise your heart rate but also make you quicker if you play any kind of stop-and-start sport. For two of these drills, you'll need to create a "ladder": Take a can of water-based spray paint out to the backyard and draw a ladder of 10 successive 18-inch squares.

Double-Leg Vertical Jumps: From a standing, one-quarter squat position, jump forward, bringing both knees toward your chest and keeping your feet together. Repeat continuously for 20 to 30 yards.

Run Throughs: From a standing start, run through the ladder, putting one foot in each box. (For a real challenge, try lifting each heel higher than the opposite knee.) Turn around at the end and repeat 6 to 8 times. Catch your breath, then do the same drill, but put two feet in each box.

Laterals: Do the ladder sideways by hopping. For the first set of 6 to 8, put one foot in each box. For the second set, put two feet in each.

The T Drill: Set cones up in the shape of T with the long stem about 10 yards long and each wing on the top of the T about 5 yards long. Starting from the bottom of the T,

---

"THANKS, ABS DIET!"

BRIAN MISHOE

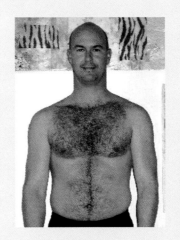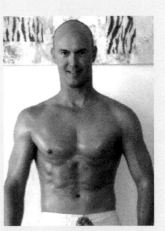

WEIGHT, WEEK 1: 174
WEIGHT, WEEK 6: 158

"The meal plan got me eating well again and boosted my metabolism, while the workout had me burning fat and building muscle. I am amazed with my results, and I know they will last because the program is so easy to follow."

ABS DIET SUCCESS STORY

"I'M SEEING DEFINITION I HAVEN'T SEEN IN YEARS"

Name: Kristen Hutchinson

Age: 39

Height: 5'4"

Starting weight: 134

Six weeks later: 124

When Kristen Hutchinson came across the Abs Diet, she was frustrated—frustrated that her running routine wasn't keeping the weight off, frustrated that she'd gained back some of the weight she'd lost on Weight Watchers, frustrated that she hadn't found the answer.

"The Abs Diet just seemed to make sense. I gave it a shot," she says, "and it was perfect."

By changing her diet with more whole grains, fruits, and vegetables (and fewer bagels) and changing her exercise program to include a quick resistance workout, Hutchinson knocked off the weight she wanted to. She also learned some new things about food. "I realized almonds are good for you. That's a treat every single day," she says.

What Hutchinson immediately noticed was the upper-body tone—especially in her shoulders and arms. It then worked its way down.

"I'm beginning to see definition in my stomach I haven't seen in years," she says.

Hutchinson especially liked the fact that the workouts are flexible in that she can go to the gym and use equipment if she wants, or do the exercises at home with dumbbells if her day becomes too busy. "I also like all the options for abs exercises," she says. "You could just modify it a little bit and not get bored. I like the variety."

Now, she appreciates the fact she's in maintenance mode and can enjoy a cheat day instead of a cheat meal. But one of the biggest rewards, she says, is that the diet reduced her back pain dramatically. She says that since starting the Abs Diet, she has very little, if any, back pain—and it's one of the many benefits she talks about when she speaks of the diet to others. Hutchinson also has a much greater energy level.

"At almost 40 years old, I feel that I have just as much energy as I did 20 years ago," she says. "In fact, because of the Abs Diet, I am now training to compete for a sprint triathlon this fall. The last one I competed in was 12 years ago. I feel that I am as in shape as I was 12 years ago because of the success of the Abs Diet.

"It's a very easy diet, and I've recommended it to so many people," Hutchinson says. "I don't even have it in my hands anymore because I've lent it to a few people so they could get the same benefit from the book that I did."

run forward, then side shuffle to the left, side shuffle all the way to the right, side shuffle back to the middle, then run backwards down the stem of the T. Rest for 30 seconds, then repeat 3 to 5 times.

The Sand-Man Interval

I know. When you're on the beach, you're looking at other people's bellies—not worrying about your own. But sand is actually one of the best surfaces for interval training because it's unstable, meaning your core really has to work hard to keep you from eating sand. Do this workout, then take a well-deserved dip.

EXERCISE	REPETITIONS	REST	SETS
SHUTTLE RUN	4 RUNS	1 MINUTE	2
SAND SKIP	5 EACH LEG	1 MINUTE	2
DIVE-BOMBERS	5–10	1 MINUTE	2
SQUAT JUMP	5	1 MINUTE	2
JUMP AND STICK	4 EACH SIDE	1 MINUTE	2
ROTATIONAL PUSHUP	6 EACH SIDE	1 MINUTE	2

ABS FACT

2-6

The number of inches you should be able to reach past your feet when stretching your hamstrings

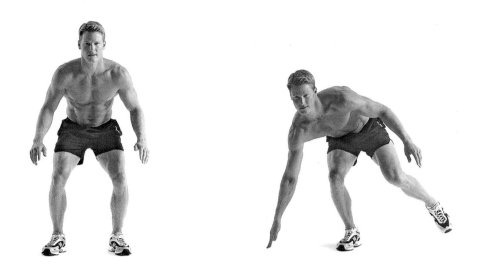

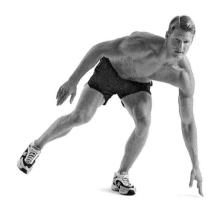

SHUTTLE RUN

Make three parallel lines in the sand, 5 yards apart. Straddle the middle line with your knees slightly bent and your elbows bent. Run to your right and reach down to touch the line with your right hand, then turn and run to the left and touch the far left line with your left hand. Then return to the middle and continue until you've completed 4 runs to each.

SAND SKIP (NOT PICTURED)

Skip forward so that you're jumping and landing on the same foot. Work on leaping as high as possible by driving your knee upward as you push off the ground with your opposite foot. Do 5 skips on each leg.

"I DROPPED MY CHOLESTEROL DRUGS"

Name: Craig Marshall

Age: 54

Height: 5'7"

Starting weight: 215

One year later: 175

In 1996, when the Olympic Torch was passing through Memphis, Craig Marshall—who was overweight and had an all-time high cholesterol level of 490—had the opportunity to be one of the torch bearers. When his wife found out, she told him, "You need to lose some weight."

So he did. Marshall went on the Atkins diet and lost 50 pounds. But the end result? He couldn't stay on it, so he gained the weight back and his cholesterol soared. Then last year, two good friends died from heart disease. "I was the pallbearer in two funerals," he says. That's when he knew he had to make a change.

"We're at Costco. My wife sees this orange cover, and we have bought every diet book, but my wife said, 'You might like this.' So I started looking at this thing and it sounded pretty good," he says. So Marshall went on the Abs Diet—revolving his diet around the Powerfoods and making good choices even while working in downtown Memphis, a hub of fried foods.

"I had my cholesterol down to 240 with medication before the diet," he says, "but now it's down to 140 and my doctor says that if it's at 140 at my next test, I can stop medication."

Marshall says he's spent more than $1,000 in clothing alterations for the 4 inches he's lost off his waist.

"Every pair of pants had to be taken in. My wife is freaking out. She asked what I'll do if I gain the weight back," Marshall says. "But after being a pallbearer at two funerals of people who were too young to die, I don't want to go back to that life. I decided to make a change in my life."

Marshall has seen his cholesterol drop and his acne clear up (since he's not eating junk anymore), and he's walking more instead of taking the trolley. Marshall, who loves the cheat meal because it gives him the opportunity to pick his poison once a week, would like to lose 20 more pounds.

"This book has been a godsend to me."

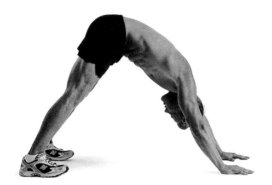

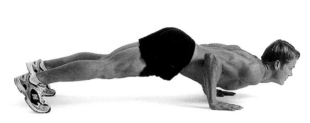

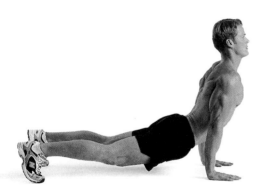

ABS FACT

30

Percentage
increase in
metabolic rate
in the hour
after drinking
17 ounces of
ice water

DIVE-BOMBERS

Put your hands and feet in the sand so your body forms an inverted V. In one fluid motion, bend your arms, sweep your upper body down and forward, and drop your butt. Then push your torso back up until your head is up, your back is arched, and your arms are straight, with your elbows locked. Hold this for a few seconds, then push back to the start. (Only your hands and toes ever touch the sand). Do 6 to 8 repetitions.

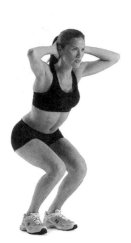
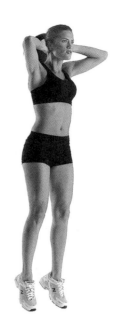

SQUAT JUMP

Stand with your feet slightly more than shoulder-width apart and your fingers laced behind your head. Bend at the knees to lower yourself until your thighs are at least parallel to the sand, then jump up as high as you can. Sink directly into the next squat without pausing. Do 6 to 8 repetitions.

ABS FACT

8

Number of days it takes your body to fully adapt to exercising in warm-weather conditions

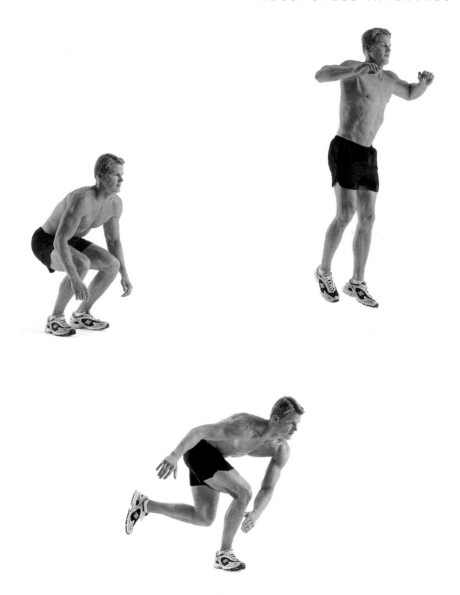

JUMP AND STICK

Stand with your feet about shoulder-width apart, hands beside your thighs. Jump straight up, then land on only one leg with your knees bent, your shoulders slightly forward, and your butt and hips back. Your hands can end up slightly out to your sides and in front of you for balance. Try to steady yourself for 2 seconds, then return to the starting position and jump again. Alternate the leg you land on and do 4 jumps on each leg.

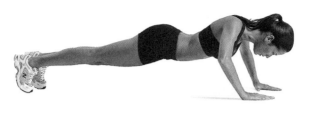

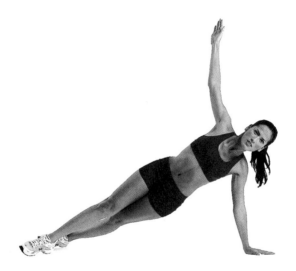

ROTATIONAL PUSHUP

Assume the classic pushup position, but as you come up, rotate your body so your right arm lifts up and extends overhead. Your arms and torso should form a T. Return to the starting position, lower yourself, then push up and rotate till your left hand points toward the sky. Do 4 to each side.

ABS DIET SUCCESS STORY

"IT'S EASY TO FIT INTO A BUSY LIFE"

Name: James Cannon

Age: 38

Height: 5'10"

Starting weight: 185

Six weeks later: 171

James Cannon was always into sports growing up. He worked out in college, then worked for 4 years in finance. That's when he decided to go to medical school.

"That left me little time for working out, so I started gaining weight—not a lot, but I became inactive," he says. "The medical profession isn't really good at taking care of itself. We tend to be overworked and don't take care of our bodies."

So along with the rigors of school and family life (he has three kids), his weight crept up. Plus, medical school didn't provide any formal training in exercise and diet.

After reading *Men's Health* magazine, Cannon decided to try the Abs Diet because it fit well with his busy lifestyle. He's been following it for a year and has maintained his 170-pound weight. He works out in the morning (so he only needs one shower a day), eats protein bars as snacks, and says his savior is a small Wendy's chili (at only 180 calories with beans and meat, it's a quick and easy snack containing several Abs Diet Powerfoods).

"A lot of people around the hospital saw the results and asked how I had the time to make the food," says Cannon, an anesthesiologist. "I told them I was really able to use the things around me, without having to make a lot of food."

Cannon has also been able to avoid his downfalls (late-night ice cream) and says the leg workout has really been a boost. "I work my legs more than I ever did. For burning fat, it's a large muscle mass that people ignore. I never really hit my legs hard. Now, if I'm going to skip a workout, it's going to be my upper body, not my legs."

Most of all, Cannon thinks it works because it gives him flexibility to make different eating choices throughout the day.

"I think it's a great plan," he says. "A lot of people at work have gone on it. It works well for a busy lifestyle."

THE ABS DIET POINT SYSTEM

ALL WORKOUTS ARE NOT MADE ALIKE. If you're currently not exercising, then anything is better than yet another *Real World* marathon. But for the most powerful workouts for burning fat and adding muscle, follow the Abs Diet Workout Worksheet.

Your goal here is to amass a total of 40 points per week. For each activity, you get full credit for doing the activity continuously for 20 minutes. Exercises in the Abs Diet Workout give you the highest number of points, but if you can't keep to that workout schedule, you can sneak in a few extra points here and there to make your workouts work. Don't try to go over 40 points though—there's no extra credit for exhaustion.

10 Points (for each 20 minutes spent)

Abs Diet Circuit

Abdominals Circuit

Interval Training (solo sport: running, swimming, cycling, machine)

6 points (for each 30 minutes spent)

Abs-specific classes

Basketball (full-court)

Boot camp classes

Boxing

Bull running, Pamplona

Calisthenics: pushups, pullups, situps

Cross-country skiing, hilly

Hiking, hilly

Hockey, inline or ice

Mountain biking, intermediate to advanced, hilly course

Pilates, advanced

Power lifting

Snowshoeing, hilly

Spinning classes

Sports-conditioning classes

Stairclimbing, stadium stairs

Strength training, noncircuit

Volleyball, beach, competitive

4 Points (for each 30 minutes spent)

Basketball, half-court

BOSU classes

Dodgeball

Inline skating, steady

Downhill skiing, intermediate to advanced

Kickboxing classes

Martial arts

Pilates, beginner

Racquetball

Rowing machine, steady

Rugby

Soccer

Step classes

Strength training, resistance bands

Strength training, ultra-light weights

Surfing

Swimming, steady

Tennis, competitive

Ultimate Frisbee

Volleyball, indoor

Yoga, advanced or power

3 Points (for every 30 minutes spent)

Adventure racing

Cross-country skiing, flat

Cycling, road, steady pace, flat

Dance-aerobic classes

Downhill skiing, easy

Fishing, big-league tuna

Golf, without cart

Hiking, flat

Jogging, steady pace

Kayaking/canoeing

Rock climbing

Snowboarding

Stairclimbing machine, steady pace

Tennis, recreational

Urban Rebounding classes

Volleyball, beach, recreational

Walking, brisk

Yoga, beginner

2 Points (for every 30 minutes spent)

Basketball, solo

Bowling

Fishing, recreational

Frisbee golf

Gardening

Golf, driving range

Golf, with cart

Ice skating, recreational

Softball

Stretching, general

Walking, slow

Water aerobic classes

Wrestling, with kids

Yoga, meditative

SHOW OFF YOUR MUSCLE

The time may come when you need your muscles for something *really* important. Here's how to prepare.

HOW TO	THE TRICK	THE BEST EXERCISE TO PREPARE FOR IT
Wrestle an alligator	It's all about speed, timing, strength, and agility. Climb onto the back of the gator, facing its head, and plant your feet behind the reptile's front legs to keep it immobilized (and if it reaches back to bite, it'll bite itself). Coming from around the side, clasp its mouth shut in one quick motion (it's not as hard as you think because the muscles it uses to open are much smaller than the ones it uses to bite). Use your other hand to wrap its mouth with duct tape.	Stationary bike. It helps you develop endurance, strength, and speed you'll need. Once you can do it comfortably for 20 minutes, increase the speed and/or resistance by 10 percent.
Drive a golf ball 300 yards	Golfing is all about rotation—so you need strong legs, abs, and back to generate the torque you need and to absorb the twists and turns of a golf swing.	The deadlift, because it hits all three of those areas. Standing with your feet about 16 inches apart, place two dumbbells on the floor—one near the outside of each foot. Bend down and grab the dumbbells with your palms facing in. Keep your knees bent, back straight, and head up. With your elbows locked, slowly straighten up, pause, then return the weights to the floor.
Rescue someone from a burning building	Forget the over-the-shoulder move—you'll bang her head on everything. Do the fireman's drag. Roll the victim on her back, get behind her, sit her up and cross her arms over her chest. Grabbing her right wrist with your left hand and her left wrist with your right, give her a big hug and lift her until she's a few feet off the floor. Now, drag her out.	One-legged press. It works the legs and shoulders and improves balance. Holding a dumbbell in each hand, stand a foot in front of a bench, facing away. With your left leg bent at 45 degrees and your toes resting on the bench for balance, slowly squat until your right thigh is nearly parallel to the floor. Return to the starting position.
Win an arm-wrestling contest	Keep your hands and shoulders as close as possible; the closer you are, the more leverage you have. And jump right after "go"—most matches are won within the first 10 seconds.	Behind-the-back wrist curls, for great forearm and wrist strength. Stand straight, holding a light barbell behind your lower back. Your hands should be about 6 inches apart, with the backs of your hands flat against your butt. With your arms straight, curl the weight up as far as you can, bending only at the wrists.

HOW TO	THE TRICK	THE BEST EXERCISE TO PREPARE FOR IT
Push a car out of the snow	Think of making a football block; the motion used to free LaDainian Tomlinson up the middle is the same one used to free your car from the blizzard.	Blocking sled. (What, you don't keep one in the garage?) Stand a few feet in front of the sled, then drop to the three-point stance: knees bent, hips lower than your head, with your head up and the fingers of your right hand on the ground. Rush forward and drive into the pads with either your forearms, shoulder, or palms. Push the sled until you've moved it 5 yards, rest 30 seconds, then do it 5 to 10 times.
Ring the bell at the state fair	You need upper-body strength, but you can get a bigger advantage by taking a few rapid, shallow breaths a few seconds before swinging. Hyper-breathing gives an adrenaline boost—as well as a boost in strength (but don't overdo it; you could faint).	Pullover, to build triceps, back, and chest muscles to raise the weight and swing down. Lie faceup on an exercise bench so the top half of your head extends past the end of the bench. Hold a single dumbbell above your chest, with the top plate resting on your palms, thumbs around the handle. Slowly lower the weight behind your head in a semicircular motion, bringing it as far down as you can without straining.
Land a 1,000-pound marlin	Keep pumping the rod in short strokes so there's no slack in the line (or else it'll turn its head and take off). And don't use your back—keep the rod close to your body and push off the footrest with your legs, sliding your butt back and forth on the chair. Hold the rod close with your biceps.	Rowing machine. It develops legs, biceps, and back—to build strength and endurance. Warm up with 12 strokes a minute for 5 minutes, then increase to 22 to 24 per minute.
Change a tire—fast	It's all about the back (to pull the tire off the axle) and the arms (to work the jack).	Bent-over dumbbell row. With your left knee on a bench and your right foot flat on the floor, hold a dumbbell in your right hand so the weight dangles as your right arm hangs down. With your back straight, pull the weight up until it touches your armpit. Slowly lower the weight to the starting position.
Hoist heavy luggage overhead	Upper back muscles will get the luggage up and shoulder muscles will get it over your head.	Military press. Standing with your feet shoulder-width apart, hold a pair of dumbbells, palms in. Slowly raise the weights to shoulder height, rotating your palms forward. Now press the weights straight above your head, stopping before you lock your elbows. Lower the weight to shoulder height.

Chapter 5

ABS DIET POWER 12

Paired with ABS3, the Abs Diet Eating Plan Will Help Build Your Body—
And Satisfy You at the Same Time

TO ME, THE REASON WHY MOST DIETS fail is math. With many diets, you have to count this, divide that, weigh this, calculate percentages, determine your zone, bust your sugar, ugh. In some of these plans, you need more math skills than a calculus scholar to figure out what you're supposed to eat and when. If you've made it this far, then you certainly know how important exercise is to reshaping your body. But if you don't eat right, you can be the most religious exerciser in the world and still look like Buddha. That's why I developed an eating plan that eliminates all the math, calculations, and square roots of Jared. I wanted it to be simple to remember and simple to follow. All you have to know is my six guidelines for a 6-pack and remember the Abs Diet Power 12 to make your eating plan as effective—and simple—as your workout plan.

Guideline 1: Eat Six Meals a Day

Most diets require that you eat less. The Abs Diet has you eating more. In fact, you *have* to eat more if you want lose more. Researchers at Georgia State University developed a technique to measure what's called "energy balance"—that is, how many calories you burn versus how many calories you take in. The researchers found that if you maintain your hourly surplus or deficit to within 300 to 500 calories at all times, you will best be able to change your body composition by losing fat and adding lean muscle mass. Subjects who added three snacks a day to three regular meals balanced out their energy better, lost fat, and increased lean body mass, as well as increased their power and endurance.

Those subjects with the largest energy imbalances (those who were over 500 calories in either ingestion or expenditure) were the fattest, while those with the most balanced energy levels were the leanest. So if you eat only three meals a day, you create imbalances in your energy levels; between meals, you're burning many more calories than you're taking in. At mealtimes, you're taking in many more than you're burning.

In a similar study, researchers in Japan found that boxers who consumed the same number of calories a day from either two or six meals both lost an average of 11 pounds in 2 weeks. But the boxers who ate six meals a day lost 3 pounds more fat and 3 pounds less muscle than the ones who ate only two meals. There's science to support the fact that more meals work, but the plain-speak reason the Abs Diet works is because it does some-

MORE FOOD = MORE MUSCLE = LESS FLAB

Yes, this an exercise guide. But to talk about exercise without discussing nutrition would be like talking about Ron Jeremy without mentioning his . . . moustache. In order for this approach to work, you must treat the two as equals: Follow the plan, see the results. In an almond shell, here's how it works. Many people have perpetuated the theory that you have to starve yourself in order to lose weight. In fact, eating less actually makes you gain fat, because your body thinks it's in starvation mode and stores fat in preparation for those times you're without food. In order to keep your metabolism revved, you need to eat—Abs Diet Powerfoods, six meals a day. That not only keeps you from feeling hungry so that you don't splurge, but it also serves the essential function of feeding your muscles so that they can grow. In short:

More food = More muscle = Less flab

Less food = Less muscle = More flab

thing that many diets don't: It keeps you full and satiated (as long as you're eating the right kinds of food), which will reduce the likelihood of a diet-destroying binge.

How it works: For scheduling purposes, alternate your larger meals with smaller snacks. Eat two of your snacks roughly 2 hours before lunch and dinner, and one snack roughly 2 hours after dinner.

Sample time schedule:

8 A.M.: breakfast

11 A.M.: snack

1 P.M.: lunch

4 P.M.: snack

6 P.M.: dinner

8 P.M.: snack

ABS FACT

600

Number of calories that people underestimate restaurant meals to be

Guideline 2: Make These 12 Abs Diet Powerfoods the Staples of Your Diet

The Abs Diet teaches you to focus on (not restrict yourself to) a handful of food types—the Abs Diet Power 12—to fulfill your core nutritional needs. These foods are all designed to boost metabolism, build muscles, and keep you away from destructive foods. Just as important, I've designed the Power 12 to include literally thousands of food combinations. There are hundreds of dairy products, fruits and vegetables, lean meats, and other choices to satisfy your tastes. Incorporating these Powerfoods into your six meals a day will satisfy your taste buds and cravings and keep you from feasting on dangerous fat promoters.

Almonds and other nuts

Beans and legumes

Spinach and other green vegetables

Dairy (fat-free or low-fat milk, yogurt, cheese)

Instant oatmeal (unsweetened, unflavored)

Eggs

Turkey and other lean meats

Peanut butter

Olive oil

Whole-grain breads and cereals

Extra-protein (whey) powder

Raspberries and other berries

How it works: Incorporate these foods into all of your meals and snacks. If you revolve your diet around them, they'll provide the nutrients your body needs, help regulate your hunger, keep you satisfied, and work to help build muscle and burn fat.

PRE- AND POST-WORKOUT SNACKS

By eating six meals a day, you'll be plenty fueled for your workouts. But a smoothie made of protein and carbohydrates about an hour before or directly after your workout can give you extra power to get through a workout or help relieve hunger afterward. For other options:

• A University of Washington study found that drinks that blend carbohydrates and protein, such as **chocolate milk,** are nearly 40 percent more effective than protein alone at helping your muscles repair themselves and grow after a workout.

• University of Florida researchers found that a combination of vitamin E, omega-3 fatty acids, and flavonoids helps muscles quickly repair after intense lifting or long runs. In a 2-week study, people who took a daily supplement containing the three compounds had 50 percent less muscle inflammation after performing arm curls than those who took a placebo. Load your diet with **fish** for omega-3s and **almonds** and **fortified cereals** for vitamin E. These nutrients need time to be absorbed, but you can have the flavonoids—try **citrus fruits, grapes, and grape juice**—right before your workout.

• Before a workout, try dry **figs** for slow-burning energy or **whole-grain toaster waffles,** which have a great blend of complex carbohydrates, fiber, protein, and unsaturated fats.

Guideline 3: Drink Smoothies Regularly

Smoothies made with a mixture of the Abs Diet Powerfoods like milk, berries, low-fat yogurt, and whey powder can act as meal substitutions and as potent snacks, and they work effectively for several reasons.

• They require little time.

• Adding berries, flavored whey powder, or peanut butter will make them taste like dessert, which will satisfy your sweet cravings.

• Their thickness takes up a lot of space in your stomach.

• Researchers at Purdue University found that people stayed fuller longer when they drank thick drinks than when they drank thin ones—even when calories, temperatures, and amounts were equal.

• A Penn State study found that men who drank yogurt shakes that had been blended until they doubled in volume ate 96 fewer calories a day than men who drank shakes of normal thickness.

• A University of Tennessee study found that men who added three servings of yogurt a day to their diets lost 61 percent more body fat and 81 percent more stomach fat over 12 weeks than men who didn't eat yogurt. Researchers speculated that the calcium helps the body burn fat and limit the amount of new fat your body can make.

How it works: Drink an 8-ounce smoothie for breakfast, as a meal substitute, or as a snack before or after your workout.

Guideline 4: Stop Counting

ABS FACT

1

Pound of muscle mass the average sedentary man loses every year

By eating these 12 Abs Diet Powerfoods and their many relatives, the foods themselves will, in a way, count your calories so you don't have to. That's because they contain a strong mix of satiating protein, healthy fats, and fiber-rich carbohydrates. Of course, that doesn't give you license to speed down the road of huge portions. A good rule: Stick to one to two servings per food group, and keep the total contents of each meal contained to the diameter of your plate. A height restriction is in effect.

ABS DIET SUCCESS STORY

"I'M ON THE ABS DIET FOR LIFE"

Name: Marian Nagel

Age: 44

Height: 5'6"

Starting weight: 148

Six weeks later: 136

As a mother of teenagers, Marian Nagel came to a point when she had to make a decision: "Do I want to be old and fat or old and healthy?"

So she decided to get back in shape for herself—as well as to inspire her son to do so, too. After purchasing *Men's Health* magazine to help him, she learned about the Abs Diet and they both tried it. She told her son, "This isn't a diet; it's a list of foods you need to eat more of." Within 6 weeks, her son dropped from 324 pounds to 292—and she dropped 12 pounds. (Since then, she has dropped down to 132, and she's now focused on losing just 4 more pounds.)

"Especially for women over 40, it gets harder and harder to lose that belly fat after having kids," says Nagel. She went from 27 percent body fat to about 20 during the initial part of the program and especially liked doing the interval training on a treadmill. "But I lost an incredible amount of inches. During the 6 weeks, I lost about 3½ inches off my waist. How nice it is to be curvy again. I see guys at the gym who can't do the abs work that I do."

Nagel also thinks the eating plan is perfect for women. "Women have a tendency to be nervous eaters more than men, and they assume they're going to eat more and take more calories if they eat six meals a day. But if you do it the proper way, you're nourishing your body, which speeds metabolism. You're eating to be sure your body is burning something all the time."

But for all the help the Abs Diet has given her, she's especially happy for the way it's helped her son.

"The best thing for me is to set an example—not only to get myself in great shape but to be a good example for him," Nagel says. "I absolutely love it, I'm still doing it—it's more of a lifestyle change than a temporary thing. I'm on the Abs Diet for life."

Guideline 5: Know What to Drink—And What Not To

Alcohol and soda add calories that you don't need right now. These empty calories don't actually help make you full or decrease the amount of food you'll eat. In fact, alcohol tempts you to eat more and encourages your body to burn less fat. When Swiss researchers gave eight healthy men enough alcohol to exceed their daily calorie requirements by 25 percent (five beers for someone who eats 3,000 calories a day), they found that booze actually impaired men's ability to burn fat by as much as 36 percent. Booze also makes you store fat. Your body sees alcohol as a poison and tries to get rid of it. So your liver stops processing all other calories until it has dealt with the alcohol. Anything else you eat while you're drinking most likely will end up as fat.

On the other hand, drinking about eight glasses of water a day has a lot of benefits. It helps keep you satiated (a lot of times what we interpret as hunger is really thirst). Water flushes the waste products your body makes when it breaks down fat for energy or when it processes protein. You also need water to transport nutrients to your muscles, to help digest food, and to keep your metabolism clicking.

How it works: I'd encourage you to stay off the booze for the 6-week plan. At the least, limit yourself to two or three alcoholic drinks per week. The best drink choices are fat-free, 1 percent, or 2 percent milk; water; and green tea (or, if you must, two glasses of diet soda a day).

EAT MORE, LOSE MORE

One of the Abs Diet principles is to eat often. A French study confirmed it: The fewer meals you eat, the more likely you are to be heavy.

NUMBER OF MEALS EATEN EACH DAY	AVERAGE BMI	WAIST-TO-HIP RATIO
1–2	28.7	0.98
3	26.2	0.95
4	26.4	0.94
5	24.5	0.93

Guideline 6: For One Meal a Week, Forget the First Five Guidelines

That's right: Cheat. For one meal a week, have whatever it is that you miss the most while you're on this plan. Have it, savor it, and then dig back in for another week. I want you to cheat for a couple reasons. One, I want *you* to control when you cheat. If you can make it through 6 days, you can reward yourself and realize that 6 days of good eating is a regimen you can stick to over the long term. And there's another important reason I want you to cheat: because it'll actually help you change your body. Researchers at the National Institutes of Health found that men who ate twice as many calories in a day as they normally did increased their metabolism by 9 percent in the 24-hour period that followed. In fact, many of the people who have succeeded on the Abs Diet credit the cheat meal as one of the greatest features of the diet—because it means that you can still enjoy all of your favorite foods without the guilt and with the extra weight. (By the way, many people say they abandon the cheat meal down the road because they find themselves actually craving the Powerfoods over the foods they used to crave!)

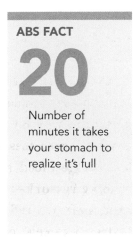

ABS FACT

20

Number of minutes it takes your stomach to realize it's full

The Abs Diet Power 12: A Recap

A   Almonds and Other Nuts/Seeds

Includes: Almonds, peanuts, walnuts, Brazil nuts, cashews, hazelnuts, pecans, pine nuts, pumpkin seeds, sunflower seeds, avocados

Why?   Nuts and some seeds contain both protein and monounsaturated fats that help you feel full. Specifically, almonds contain magnesium—a key component in muscle building.

Doesn't include: Smoked and salted nuts

Tip: Eat about 24 almonds—or two handfuls—a day. One study showed that, even with the higher fat content, eating that amount didn't lead to weight gain. That amount should also suppress your appetite, so it's a good late-afternoon snack. You can also sneak nuts in smoothies, over cereal, or sliced on a side dish of broccoli.

"I ADJUSTED THE ABS DIET TO MY NEEDS"

Name: Ken Roberts

Age: 35

Height: 5'7½"

Starting weight: 165

Six weeks later: 150

Starting body-fat percentage: 18 percent

Six weeks later: 13.8 percent

Ken Roberts is the typical yo-yo. He'd be in shape and have a 6-pack for a year or so, then something would throw him off—a holiday season, getting married, losing a job, a hankering for root beer floats. "But usually the thing that kicks me in the ass is my back acts up. With an 18-month-old and another on the way, it's a big motivation to get in shape, because somebody has to bring them up the stairs," he says.

So Roberts went on the Abs Diet—with one big adjustment. Lactose intolerant, he wasn't able to use many dairy products. So he subbed in soy milk with oatmeal and used cottage cheese instead of yogurt. Then he added a very easy workout program—resistance exercise 3 days a week and some treadmill work. "The diet was key," he says. Now, he cheats on cheat days, but not too much.

"During my wife's last pregnancy, she's eating and I'm eating. This time around, as she's getting bigger, I'm getting smaller."

But Roberts says he has the biggest motivator of all—being able to be active with his children.

"Millions of Americans have chronic back pain. I don't want to be part of that group," he says. "I don't want to fall back the next holiday season or when the next baby is born."

B   Beans and Legumes

Includes: Soy beans, pinto beans, chickpeas (garbanzo beans), navy beans, black beans, white beans, kidney beans, lima beans, green beans, lentils, peas, hummus, edamame

Why?   They're packed with protein, iron, and fiber, which help you both build muscle and lose weight.

Doesn't include: Refried beans (high in saturated fat) or baked beans (high in sugar)

Tip: Sub black beans for ground beef in meat-heavy dishes to eliminate saturated fats and add fiber.

S   Spinach and Other Green Vegetables

Includes: Spinach, broccoli, Brussels sprouts, asparagus, peppers, some lettuces

Why?   Green vegetables, particularly spinach, have the vitamin power to protect you against heart disease and stroke. Broccoli is loaded with calcium and vitamin C.

Doesn't include: Iceberg lettuce (contain no vitamins, minerals, and little fiber, unlike other kinds of lettuce, like romaine or arugula)

Tip: Don't like veggies? Mask them in chili, or add a few to a chicken stir-fry made with olive oil and garlic.

D   Dairy, Fat-Free or Low-Fat

Includes: Milk, yogurt, cheese, cottage cheese

Why?   Calcium has been shown to be a key ingredient in weight loss. Used as a base for smoothies, low-fat milk helps give smoothies volume to keep your stomach full and you satisfied.

Doesn't include: Whole milk (high in fat), frozen yogurt (high in sugar)

Tip: Drink a glass of 2 percent milk before dinner to help take up some room in your stomach. Make an instant (and guilt-free) dessert with a small scoop of chocolate powder added to a glass of low-fat milk.

I   Instant Oatmeal, Unsweetened, Unflavored

Includes: Other high-fiber cereals

Why?   Oatmeal contains soluble fiber, which helps lower your cholesterol. In one study, oatmeal was shown to sustain your blood sugar levels longer than many other foods. That ensures you won't be ravenous for several hours afterwards and that you'll keep your metabolism fast.

Doesn't include: Oatmeal with sugar or high-fructose corn syrup

Tip: Add a little cooked oatmeal to a smoothie for increased fiber. Nuke oatmeal with frozen berries and 1 percent milk for a good after-dinner snack.

E   Eggs

Includes: Eggs, egg whites

Why?   The protein found in eggs is more effective for building muscle than protein from other sources. Increasingly, research shows that eating an egg or two a day won't raise your cholesterol levels.

Doesn't include: The "everything" omelet at the local diner

Tip   Need a fast breakfast? Mix two eggs in a bowl and nuke them for 60 to 90 seconds: instant scrambled eggs.

T   Turkey and Other Lean Meats

Includes: Turkey, chicken, fish (especially salmon and tuna), shellfish, Canadian bacon, lean steak like extra-lean ground beef, tenderloin, London broil, flank steak

Why?   Since your body uses more energy to digest protein than it does to digest carbohydrates or fat, you're burning more calories simply by eating protein. But protein also helps build muscle and keep you replete. The best tactic is to split your primary meat choices between fish and poultry, with occasional portions of red meat. Fish is loaded with polyunsaturated fats, and chicken and turkey have the lean protein to build muscle.

Doesn't include: Sausage, bacon, cured meats, ham, fatty cuts of steak

Tip: Don't like fish? Eat flaxseed—ground or oil. One teaspoon has only 60 calories, but it contains 4 grams of fiber and is loaded with omega-3s. You can find both in most health food stores. Sprinkle in oatmeal or in smoothies.

P   Peanut Butter

Includes: Peanut butter, all-natural and sugar-free; almond butter

Why?   It contains monounsaturated fats, which have been shown to help keep you full, and it's also one of those sinful-tasting foods that help add variety and taste to a diet.

Doesn't include: Sugary brands or trans fatty peanut butters

Tip: Limit yourself to 3 tablespoons a day because of its high fat content. A perfect snack: PB on whole-wheat toast with crushed berries.

O   Olive Oil

Includes: Olive oil, canola oil, peanut oil, sesame oil

Why?   With the same monounsaturated fats as peanut butter, it'll help you control cravings.

ABS DIET SUCCESS STORY

"IT HELPED ME HANDLE STRESS"

Name: Casey Getz

Age: 28

Height: 5'10"

Starting weight: 184

Six weeks later: 168

When Casey Getz lost his job, the stress started and the healthy living ended.

"I got to the point where I looked at my stomach and said, 'I've got to do something about this now,'" he says.

After reading about the Abs Diet, the first thing he did was buy the 12 Powerfoods and join the local gym. He followed the recommended Powerfoods—and then added his own twist. He counted calories to ensure that he was eating 300 fewer calories than he needed every day. (The Abs Diet doesn't require—or even want—you to count calories, but some people do find it effective for keeping track of what they eat.) He ate every 3 hours—and really leaned heavily on salmon, beans, and almonds. "I'd grab a handful of almonds when I started to get hungry. You don't always have the time to make a meal, and almonds really satisfied me until the next meal," he says.

"Right away, just switching to those foods worked," Getz says. "I dropped 4 pounds the first week and then consistently 2 pounds a week after that."

Now, he's in a maintenance pattern. He's got a marathon in his sights, he has extra confidence in his ability to eat healthy at any time, and he's got more oomph for handling the stresses of graduate school.

"Now I feel like I've got an extra battery," Getz says. "That's for all aspects of life, whether studying, working, or home. You've got an extra reserve if you're eating like that."

Doesn't include: Vegetable oil and hydrogenated vegetable oils, trans fatty acids, margarine

Tip: To integrate some into your meals, drip a little on vegetables, salad, even rice or a baked potato.

W   Whole-Grain Bread and Cereals

Includes: Whole-grain bread, whole-grain cereal, brown rice, whole-wheat pretzels, whole-wheat pasta

Why? "Whole-grain" means that the unrefined parts of the product that contain important nutrients and fiber remain. All-white breads and pastas don't contain those fiber-rich elements that help your digestive system. Whole-grain foods keep your insulin levels low, so you're less likely to store fat.

Doesn't include: White bread, bagels, doughnuts, breads labeled as "wheat" instead of "whole wheat"

Tip: Buy whole-wheat pasta with flaxseed for a double-punch of power. It not only tastes good but is also nutritionally superior to regular pasta.

E   Extra-Protein (Whey) Powder

Includes: Whey powder, ricotta cheese

Why? Whey protein is a high-quality protein that contains amino acids, which build muscle and burn fat; it has the highest amount of protein for the fewest number of calories

Doesn't include: Soy protein

Tip: Drink a smoothie with whey before a workout. One study found that it helped increase lifters' ability to build muscle compared to those lifters who drank one after working out.

R   Raspberries and Other Berries

Includes: Raspberries, blueberries, blackberries, strawberries, cranberries, and other fruits like apples

Why? Berries are powerful sources of cancer-fighting antioxidants, but they also contain fiber to keep you fuller longer.

Doesn't include: Jelly

Tip: Want the most powerful berry? Pick blueberries—they're tops in antioxidants and they're loaded with soluble fiber.

ABS FACT

10

Pounds you would gain by skipping breakfast for a year

HE GOT FIT, HE'S STAYING FIT
Let His Story Inspire You to Make the Abs Diet Part of Your Life

KYLE SNAY HAS DROPPED NEARLY 40 POUNDS on the Abs Diet. He was a Top 10 finisher in the initial Abs Diet Challenge. And he's been about as active in the Abs Diet phenomenon as anyone; he ran his own message board, helping other people discover what he found on the Abs Diet: success. Here's his story, in his words:

"I'm recommending physical therapy. But if you lost some weight that would help a lot."

That's what my doctor told me when my back went out on me last summer. I was 35 years old, 6-foot-5, 230 pounds, and my body was a life-sized Jell-O mold. I had been diagnosed with a herniated disc about 7 years earlier, and every now and then I'd have a major flare-up that felt like someone was using my lower back as a drill press.

I knew I had to lose weight, get back into shape, and stop two-spooning a half-gallon of ice cream in front of the TV (I didn't bother with bowls since I'd eat the entire half-gallon in one episode of *The West Wing*). Trying to keep up with my 2-year-old son was taking its toll, and my daughter was due to be born in a few months. I think everyone has a point where they say, "Screw it, I've had enough of feeling like crap." For me, it was when I left the doctor's office and added everything up—besides, I didn't want to go broke with copayments to the "physical terrorist."

On the way home, I stopped by the bookstore and began researching books on dieting.

I had never been on a diet before, but I knew I didn't have the patience or tolerance to count carbs, points, or spend 12 weeks living off grapefruit. I didn't find anything close to encouraging so I grabbed an issue of *Men's Health* magazine on the way out for inspiration. That night while reading it in bed (after polishing off an entire box of Little Debbie cake rolls), I came across the introductory article on the Abs Diet program and everything *clicked*.

Here was a plan that combined exercise with a nutrition program based on common-sense eating guidelines. I couldn't believe how organized it was, and yet at the same time it seemed very flexible and easy to follow. I told my wife that I had found my plan for getting back into shape. She didn't seem too convinced, since I had failed several times before over the past 10 years at the cost of numerous gym memberships. But the difference this time was that I had a plan and a lot of motivation (it's not a pretty picture when you look more pregnant than your wife who's due to give birth in a couple of months).

I still had to wait a couple of weeks before I could get my hands on the book, so I used the time to take a hard look at my capabilities. I didn't think the food would be a problem, especially since I could eat six meals a day. But I had to be realistic about the workout, mainly because I had blown too many attempts by being unmotivated and lazy. I work at a university and have access to the weight room, but with a hectic work schedule and my free time becoming nearly nonexistent once the baby arrived, I decided to purchase a home gym. I knew that my workout times would have to be early in the morning, so I needed the flexibility of a home gym in case I missed a session and needed to make it up without leaving the house. I had the room for a gym in my basement, and after a lot of research I found one that met my needs. The store I was buying it from was having a promotion where they were giving away a free recumbent bike with the purchase, so that took care of my cardio program as well.

Needless to say, my wife was not exactly on board with the idea. I had cashed in a small retirement account to purchase the gym, and with a baby on the way, our budget was extremely tight. In a nutshell, I had fully committed myself to getting into shape or facing the wrath of a hormonally imbalanced pregnant woman who had access to the kitchen knives while I slept.

But seriously, I knew it was now or never. I had a family to support and I needed to be there for them and take responsibility for my health in order to do so.

I started the Abs Diet during the first week of August. I didn't know what to expect since I hadn't been on a diet before. In high school and in college, I had lifted quite a bit, so I wasn't unfamiliar with weight training. During the first week, I thought I was going to rupture an artery on several occasions. I had decided to start off doing all three circuits in the circuit routine and high-intensity interval training sessions for my cardio. It was definitely the toughest week of my life. The diet was going well, though. My wife was extremely supportive and helped prepare the meals and keep me on track.

While I would have traded a kidney for a cupcake, I ate clean that week for the first time in my life, and it felt great. At the end of the first week I had lost 7 pounds. I decided to hold off another week before taking another photo to compare to my "before shot." By that time, I had lost a total of 10 pounds. Taking photos every 2 weeks was probably the best thing I did for feedback. When you look at yourself every day in the mirror, you don't notice the changes that your body is going through, but the photos spoke volumes. I could definitely see a change in my body, and I noticed that my clothes were fitting a little looser. Two weeks later, I had lost another 10 pounds and people were starting to take notice. My belt was on its last notch and I had energy that wasn't there a month ago. That week my daughter was born, and I couldn't believe how different my face looked in the photos with her. The diet was going great. My job kept me busy and I had no time to think about being distracted with cheating. I even purchased a handheld blender and a small fridge that I kept in my office to make smoothies.

At the end of 6 weeks, I had lost another 2 pounds. I had actually dropped that during the fifth week. I was looking at a different person in my "after photo." I couldn't believe my new body and the bells and whistles that came with it. Fall was approaching, and I had to replace my entire cold-weather wardrobe because none of my clothes from the previous winter fit. I knew that I would never go back to being the same person I was before beginning the Abs Diet. I had become an inspiration to friends and family. The opportunity to help others who were in my situation was extremely rewarding.

It's been nearly 9 months since I started the Abs Diet and I'm just as dedicated as I was during the first week. I change my workout every couple of months and even did the circuit routine again to help a buddy of mine who was looking to lose weight. During that time, I dropped down from 230 pounds to 192 pounds, and since then I've significantly increased my muscle mass.

I've learned that the diet was never a diet, but simply a lifelong plan for eating and living healthy. Over the past 9 months I've never missed a workout and I've yet to step foot inside a fast food restaurant. But this doesn't mean that I don't enjoy food. Every weekend I eat whatever I want and savor every bite without worrying about going overboard. It's the best of both worlds.

It took 35 years to realize it, but only 6 weeks to experience it. I'll be forever grateful to the Abs Diet and what it's done for me.

Oh yeah, I never did make that physical therapy appointment for my back, either.

Appendix

EXERCISE FAQS

There are a lot of people at the gym when I work out. This makes the circuit routine difficult because of the short rest time between exercises. What should I do when I'm at a crowded gym?

Take advantage of the flexibility that's built into the circuit routine. For example, you can use dumbbell exercises on benches for many exercises (so you don't have to wait in line for machines). Focus more on the muscle groups instead of the specific exercises. Remember, this guide gives you the tools and options to swap in different exercises for various body parts. In other words, have backup exercises for the same muscle group in place in case the machine for your primary exercise isn't available.

I occasionally have to travel for work. What can I do to get a good workout and stay in shape when I'm on the road?

If the hotel doesn't have a fitness room, some hotels offer discounted day passes to local gyms/clubs. You may also want to look at investing into a set of elastic bands (see the Band-Aid Workout, page 147), or do a workout using your own body weight (see page 104).

As for food, you can pack items that travel well. A handheld blender makes quick smoothies and will take up little space in a suitcase. You can also pack items such as protein powder, ground flaxseed, and nonfat powdered milk into sealable storage bags and make Powerfoods for any meal.

Is there a recommended pace at which I should be doing reps?

The main thing is that you don't want to use momentum to lift a weight. Use a slow, controlled speed. You can use the 2-second up, 2-second down rule, or for an even better burn, try the 2-second up and 4-second down rule; going slower on the lowering movement helps build muscle when it stresses the muscle in the "negative" position—the position when it's not trying to raise the weight, but rather trying to hold and steady it as you lower it.

Are free weights always better than machines?

Sometimes machines can build muscle better—for instance, when you need to isolate specific muscles after an injury, or when you're too inexperienced to perform a free-weight exercise. But as you become more trained, free weights should make up the major portion of your training program because they generally activate more muscle mass.

How often should I change my weight-training routine?

The only rule I have: Change when you stop seeing results—or get bored. That generally falls into the 4-to-6-week category.

I heard that lifting really slowly builds big muscles. Is that true?

Lifting super slowly produces superlong workouts—and that's it. University of Alabama researchers recently studied two groups of lifters doing a 29-minute workout. One group performed exercises using a 5-second up phase and a 10-second down phase, the other a more traditional approach of 1 second up and 1 second down. The faster group burned 71 percent more calories and lifted 250 percent more weight than the slow lifters.

I don't always feel sore after my workout. Does this mean I'm not training hard enough?

Muscle soreness after a workout is often referred to as Delayed Onset Muscle Soreness (DOMS). Many old-time bodybuilders followed the no-pain-no-gain principle, believing that if they weren't really sore the day after a workout then they hadn't lifted hard

FAT KILLS

Being overweight does more than keep the fast-food industry rich. It also can kill you. As you get heavier, the risk gets greater. Here, see how many years get knocked off your life—based on your age and BMI (body mass index; see Chapter 1).

AGE	20	30	40	50	60
YOUR BMI		YEARS OFF YOUR LIFE			
25	0	0	0	0	0
26	1	0	0	0	0
27	1	1	0	0	0
28	1	1	0	0	0
29	1	1	1	0	0
30	1	1	1	0	0
31	2	2	1	1	0
32	2	2	2	1	1
33	3	2	2	1	1
34	3	3	2	1	1
35	3	3	3	2	1
36	4	3	3	2	2
37	4	4	3	2	2
38	5	4	4	3	2
39	5	5	4	3	2
40	6	5	4	3	2
41	6	6	5	4	3
42	7	6	5	4	3
43	7	6	6	4	3
44	8	7	6	5	3
45+	13	11	10	7	5

enough. But research has shown that DOMS is not a prerequisite for muscle growth. Muscle soreness is simply the result of the damage done to muscle fibers during a challenging weight-lifting workout. Basically, when you lift a weight, small tears occur within the muscle tissues being used. When you first begin lifting weights or you change to a different routine, you will almost certainly experience some muscle soreness. This is fine, as long as you're not in so much pain that it makes you stop wanting to work out. Your body will adjust quickly, especially if you're already experienced with weight training.

How much protein do I need to eat to build muscle?

If you're working out hard, consuming more than 0.9 to 1.25 grams of protein per pound of body weight is a waste. Excess protein breaks down into amino acids and nitrogen, which are either excreted or converted into carbohydrates and stored. More important when you consume protein is that you have the right balance of carbohydrates with it. Have a post-workout shake of three parts carbohydrates and one part protein.

Index

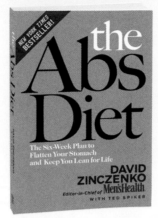
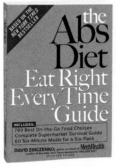
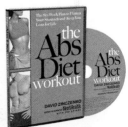